The Vitamin & Mineral HOAX

Rip-Offs and Lies at Your Expense

The Ultimate Resource Guide for Choosing Vitamins and Minerals that Nutritional Supplement Manufacturers Don't Want You to Read!

By Gregory S. Ellis, PhD, CNS

The Vitamin and Mineral Hoax:
Rip-Offs and Lies at Your Expense

The Ultimate Resource Guide for Choosing Vitamins and Minerals
that Nutritional Supplement Manufacturers Don't Want You to Read!

By Gregory S. Ellis, PhD, CNS

Published by:
Targeted Body Systems Publishing
68 Skyline Drive
Glen Mills, PA 19342
orders@TargetedBodySystems.com
610-459-3037

Printed in the United States of America

ISBN 0-9705832-0-6

Table of Contents

chapter 1

Introduction

Are you confused? You want to take a daily nutritional supplement, but you have no idea where to turn for accurate information. I see it every day in my nutritional consultation practice: clients come to my office dragging boxes and bags full of an endless array of nutritional supplements. But, here's the rub: they haven't the slightest idea about whether or not the products they purchased are of any value.

Supplement users have little idea about how to read the label on a nutritional supplement. They don't know what RDA and RDI mean, they are unable to decipher anything about the ingredients in the product, and they do not have the necessary knowledge about nutritional supplements to tell if a product contains all the nutrients they require each day. Further, they are unable to evaluate whether the nutrients contained in the capsules or tablets come from the best sources of raw ingredients and if those ingredients are blended into the product in the correct amounts and in the right balance to one another.

Well, for you dear reader, that's about to change!

You may think that choosing a nutritional supplement for your daily use, one that provides you with all the essential nutrients that you may not receive from your diet, is an easy task. It's not—far from it. There are hundreds of supplement manufacturers and thousands of supplements.

Anyone with enough money to manufacture a product is, literally, in the nutritional supplement business. Knowledge. Understanding. Experience. Forget it. Not required, not needed. If there's a buck to be made, they'll make it at your expense—at both the expense of your hard-earned dollars and, in the worst case, at the expense of your health.

You may think that companies who sell nutritional supplements know what they're doing. Most don't. That's a fact. Very few of the products sold on the market really provide you with what you need.

What they do is take the money out of your wallet. What they don't do is provide you with the return on your investment that you believe you are receiving.

OK, so you figure you'll ask a health care professional such as your medical doctor, chiropractor, or registered dietician. Forget it! It's a waste of time. Few of them had training in nutritional supplementation. Sure, they have more knowledge than you do about diseases and disease diagnosis, but most often, not about diet and supplements or about prevention of disease. And, their knowledge may even be dangerous to your health.

Magazines. Nah. Just some hack writer pounding away at his computer keyboard, re-writing thoughts and ideas he read about in some other magazine that that guy had read about in yet another magazine.

Now, take a guess. Whom do most health practitioners rely on for nutritional supplement information? The answer: the supplement manufacturer. And, as I already told you, this is a business; whoever has enough money to play, can play.

It's just like the pharmaceutical industry. Who do you think educates the medical doctors about drugs? The detail salesman from the drug company, that's who! Surprised? You shouldn't be. It's a business, a big dollar business. Don't let anyone tell you otherwise. And, the nutritional supplement industry, just like the drug business, is a business too. One with high profits and a through-the-roof growth cycle.

Today, as I write this, news of the herb revolution's arrival appeared on the cover of Time magazine. It was the lead story. Who's the newest kid on the block to join the party and the high profit growth stream? It's the big pharmaceutical houses: Bayer, Warner Lambert, Centrum. Their ads are all over TV. Where do they place the products? K-Mart, Rite-Aid, and CVS, etc.

And what's the name of game? Shelf space. And what's the financial deal? You can't get shelf space unless you meet the bottom line. At this point, it's all about pennies: not dimes, not dollars—just pennies. The cheapest product with the largest national marketing plan designed to touch the most eyes and ears possible.

If a product manufacturer wants his product on the retail shelf, he is obligated to run a TV infomercial, obligated to buy space ads in major magazines, and obligated to promote the product with his big bucks. This is the only way he can crawl-in-bed with the big boys, a.k.a. the giant marketing and distribution conglomerates. Otherwise, he's out of luck, and only the guys with the deep pockets walk in the door. It's a business of whom-do-you-know and deep pockets.

chapter 2   History of Nutritional Supplements

The minute the supplement is mass marketed, forget it: the quality and truth-in-advertising is gone. The product is half-baked, a glimmer of what it should be.

Do supplements work? Do they contribute to your health? Sure they do. But, and this is a big BUT—you've got to know what you're doing and you must know whom you can listen to. And, you must be a knowledgeable consumer. You must understand what you want and *need* (emphasis added to the word *need*) and then how to find it in the product you purchase.

This monograph will first outline key milestones in the history of the nutritional supplement industry. From that point I will build on your knowledge base and teach you the ins and outs of nutritional supplements. After a brief reading time, you'll have the necessary facts and the essential information you need to evaluate the products that you want and *need* to buy.

There are thousands of products on the market. Which ones should you buy, and which ones should you reject? That is the purpose of this monograph. Your wallet and your health depend on it.

In 1912, Dr. Casimir Funk, a nutritional research scientist, found a chemical substance in rice hulls that cured a crippling and killing disease called beriberi. The chemical he discovered, and then extracted from the rice plant, is the vitamin we now know as Vitamin B1 (thiamine). This discovery was the key scientific event that heralded the dawning of the age of nutritional science.

In 1928, Dr. Albert Szent-Gyorgyi discovered Vitamin C. Dr. Roger Williams, in 1938, found a solution to organ failure and sudden death in nutrient-depleted animals with his discovery of pantothenic acid (Vitamin B5). As we approached 1950, agriculture schools throughout the US had studied the effects of nutrient deficient diets on the health of animals. Other scientists had completed human studies to help them understand the effects of poor diets.

The influence and scientific output from these efforts were enormous. In fact, so much data had been accumulated during these years that no new vitamin has been officially recognized since 1952. Yet, the scientific work-pace today increases exponentially. It is fueled by rapid increases in technological capability, including diagnostic equipment and basic scientific methodology such as molecular biology.

The main driving force, however, is the phenomenal interest in nutrition by the public. Some estimates show that close to 50% of the people in the US use nutritional supplements. The dollar volume in sales of supplements increased from $3.4 billion in 1994 to $6.5 billion in 1998. Bean counters who follow the nutritional supplement industry predict sales of $14 billion per year by 2001-2004. There appears to be no end in sight for this startling growth curve.

But, with the growth of the industry and interest in nutritional supplements, one also realizes the growth of another aspect of nutrition-al supplementation: *confusion*. The consumer is overwhelmed by an enormous number of choices from a multitude of different supplements, including herbs, vitamins, minerals, specialized nutrients, and a wild proliferation of countless so-called disease-curing nutrients. Nutrients from this latter group are the ones touted, primarily by multi-level mar-keting companies, as the next miracle products—the ones that will cure you of everything from sniffles to cancer and heart disease. Folks, it just ain't true.

This monograph will guide you through the maelstrom of nutri-tional choices and separate fact from fiction. I will provide you with the basics of nutritional supplementation so that you can make the right choices when selecting the products you need to use regularly.

Overview of Nutrients:
Essential Nutrients versus Nutraceuticals

Before developing a detailed outline of nutritional supplemen-tation, I will define two specific groups of supplements available in the marketplace. The first group is the **essential vitamins and minerals**: these are the nutrients we must derive from our diet each day or often enough to prevent too low an intake to meet our needs. If we don't ingest them, we suffer health consequences.

This group includes all the vitamins and minerals established as essential and necessary to human health. It also includes several nutrients that, at this time, are considered provisionally necessary: that

4

is a fancy way of saying that scientists think you may need them, but they just aren't sure yet. The number of nutrients in the group I call **essential vitamins and minerals** includes about 30 different nutrients.

The second group comprises those supplements for which we have no known need: if we don't eat foods containing them or swallow a pill containing them, little damage occurs to our body. The bulk of the available supplements on the market today include items from this group. The complete herbal pharmacy provides an example of this and includes such herbs as ginseng, ginkgo, echinacea, and St. John's Wort.

A new name has developed over the last several years to describe the nutrients in this group: *nutraceutical*. The rapid growth of interest in nutrition spawned the exploding arena of Alternative Medicine in the late 1980's. A key component to the therapeutics used by Alternative Medicine specialists is nutritional supplements and, for the most part, therapeutic emphasis is on the use of the dizzying array of nutraceutical supplements. In other words, the practitioner prescribes a nutrient that may provide drug-like actions, but doesn't possess the side effects of drugs.

A notion that underpins the therapeutic use of nutritional supplements and nutraceuticals is that the body is deficient in a specific nutrient or, simultaneously, that the use of the nutrient may be blocked from incorporation into some metabolic pathway. The idea is that if restoration of the full activity of the metabolic pathway could occur as a result of supplementation with a specific nutrient, either in super-high dosages or in combination with other nutrients, then health would improve.

The body is able to manufacture its own supply of many of the nutrients now sold by manufacturers as supplemental nutraceuticals, provided that it has all the *essential* nutrients required to serve as building blocks for the newly synthesized chemicals. Examples of nutraceuticals that show great promise in providing nutritional support for the body are lipoic acid and Co-enzyme Q_{10} (CoQ10).

The primary purpose of this monograph is not an exposition of the burgeoning nutraceutical market—which should be a secondary and minor concern for you.

Its goal is to provide you with the guidelines you need to choose a supplement that you can use each day to meet your *essential* nutritional needs. The use of nutraceuticals is not of primary importance, and one should only consider using nutraceuticals *after* committing to follow a supplement program that provides all of the essential nutrients in the proper balance and formulated with the most effective raw ingredients.

In this monograph I will tell you:

• Why you should use nutritional supplements

• What specific, essential nutrients you need

• How to balance the nutrients so that you aren't ingesting too much of one and too little of another

• How much of the product listed on the label you really need—
are you getting too much or too little

• How to determine whether the <u>source</u> of the nutrient listed on the label is high-quality and readily absorbed by the body

• How to read a label and understand whether the manufacturer is giving you what you are paying for.

Many scientists believe that our diet should provide us with all the nutrients we need each day. Others argue vehemently against the "diet is enough to meet your needs" pundits. I agree with those who support supplementation.

chapter 3

Why Use
Nutritional Supplements

The United States Department of Agriculture published its findings about people's average, daily nutrient intakes in its publication the Nationwide Food Consumption Survey. This dietary analysis indicates that many men, women, and children do not meet the recommended guidelines for daily minimum nutrient intake from their diets.

The following graph illustrates the significant lack of nutrient intake in the diets of women, ages 19-50.

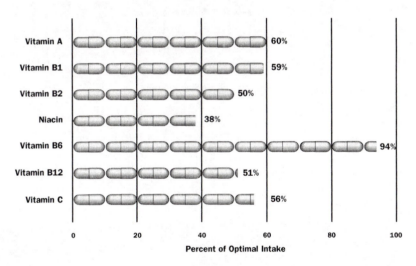

Graph 1. The 100% line is the Recommended Daily Intake (RDI) for intake of nutrients. Intakes below 75% are dangerous. The graph shows the average, daily intake for important essential nutrients as a percentage of the RDI. The average intake for many nutrients is below both the RDI and the danger point.

Data published in the early 1990's by the USDA Continuing Survey of Food Intake show similar results. Even with all the emphasis on good eating, there has been no improvement in nutrient intake from the first food intake studies completed in 1968. Low nutrient intake is as much a problem today as it was 30 years ago.

The following graph shows the low mineral intake by adults.

Low Mineral Intake by Adults

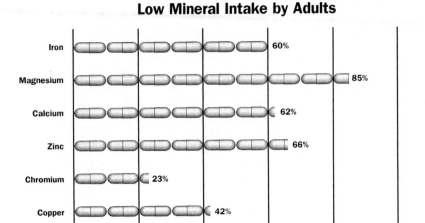

Average % Intake for Adults

- Iron 60%
- Magnesium 85%
- Calcium 62%
- Zinc 66%
- Chromium 23%
- Copper 42%
- Manganese 82%

Graph 2. The nutrient intake is compared to the US Recommended Daily Intake (RDI) except for copper and chromium, which are compared to the standard called Estimated Safe and Adequate Daily Dietary Intake (ESADDI). Note that these values are for the average amounts in the diets. By definition, this means that 49% of people eat less than the percent listed!

Only 3% of the population eats the recommended number of servings from the four food groups.

That's right! In a study by Crocetti and Guthrie, only 3% of 21,500 people ate the recommended levels of foods from the four food groups. Instead of the four servings of fruits and green vegetables per day recommended by the USDA, Americans eat an average of 0.68 servings of fruit and 0.65 servings of vegetables per day. These figures, startling in themselves, are important when you realize the amount of apparent under-nutrition for a large part of the population.

Does your diet fit these patterns? If so, you should work toward healthier eating habits. And nutritional supplements will help meet nutrient intake recommendations.

Pure Food is Poor Food

Five of the twelve leading causes of death in the United States are directly or partly nutritional in origin—cancer, heart disease, high blood pressure, diabetes, and liver disease. Trace metals such as zinc, copper, chromium, manganese, iron, calcium, and magnesium are involved in all five. A lack of dietary nutrients accounts for nearly 94% of the fatal diseases in this country (Dr. Henry Schroeder, The Poisons Around Us).

Another difficulty with modern foods is that many of them are refined. Refining was developed as a method to preserve shelf life. The purpose of refining was economic; is that a surprise?

When a food is highly refined, and the micronutrients are largely removed, the calories are called "empty," i.e., lacking in nutrients. Sugar—white sugar—is an example. It has essentially no vitamins and no minerals. But, the vitamins and minerals that were removed are necessary for the metabolism of the sugar itself. The body cannot properly break the sugar down into energy without the associated micronutrients. And those nutrients are also essential for health.

How can you be healthy if you do not ingest what the body needs?

So, sugar has no vitamins, minerals, fats, or proteins in it—it is just pure, adulterated, 99.9% refined, good-tasting carbohydrate. It unbalances the diet. Today, sugar or some new-fangled technological substitutes, such as maltodextrin or high fructose corn syrup, make up 30-40% of the daily calorie intake for many people. Many youngsters consume more than 50% of their daily calories as nutrient-depleted carbohydrates (sugar).

How can they be healthy if they do not ingest the essential nutrients?

Other carbohydrates, when refined, especially the grains and cereals, also unbalance the diet. Table 1 lists the percent of nutrients removed when foods are refined.

Nutrients Lost in the Refining of Whole Foods (%)

Nutrient	Wheat flour	Sugar, refined	Rice	Corn Starch	Milk, fat-free
Calcium	60				
Phosphorous	71				
Magnesium	85	98	83	97	6
Chromium	40	93	75	72	50
Manganese	86	89	45	93	100
Iron	76				
Cobalt	89	95	38	37	
Copper	68	83	26	31	
Zinc	78	98	75	91	14
Molydenum	48	100			90
Selenium	16	100		100	88
Vitamin B6	72	100	69	87	

Table 1.

Measured vitamin losses from refining grain show an 86% loss for vitamin E, 72-81% for the B vitamin family, 50% for the B vitamin pantothenic acid, and 67% for folic acid. The residue, know as millfeed, goes to livestock and poultry as rich vitamin and mineral supplements.

When we fractionate milk, it loses most of its manganese, molybdenum, selenium, and half of its chromium. It loses vitamins A, D, and E. The fat-free milk that is left—the skim milk, the type most people drink nowadays—still contains the magnesium, cobalt, copper, and zinc from the original whole milk. But now, nonetheless, the fat-free milk is unbalanced; it's *nutritionally incomplete*. To balance it means that we must return the butter to it. Or what is better and cheaper, throw it out and use whole milk.

Now, at this point you may cry out against the dangers of milk, but I don't want to go off into that argument. Suffice it to say that milk is almost a perfect food and will improve the health of anyone who drinks it.

A diet with plenty of white bread (including the new "perfect" food of the 1990's—bagels), refined cereals, white rice, and sugar supplies more than 40% of most people's daily calories. Sandwiches, pies, rolls, and pastry supply only 30-40% of the necessary nutrients we need each day. This diet is unbalanced and lacking. It is not healthy.

It's not a good situation and it is very hard to cover these deficiencies by diet alone. How can you meet your needs for nutrient intake?

Here's the picture: Your diet of 2,500 calories per day contains an average amount of refined sugar, similar to what most people eat today (750 calories of the total 2,500 comes from refined sugar). You also eat 800 calories per day of white flour (refined bread, cereals, baked goods, pizza, and cookies). Seventy percent of the 800 calories that you ingest as white flour each day are empty, i.e., devoid of nutrients.

To meet your needs, you will have to fill your daily intake of 1,310 "empty" calories, i.e., calories having no nutritional value with 24 nutrients from other sources (750 from sugar and 70% of 800 calories from refined grains = 560 calories). Where will you get them?

There is another problem, and it's significant. The figure of 2,500 calories, as a daily intake of total calories for most people, is much too high. That was years ago. Due to the low level of physical activity of most people, the average caloric intake for women is about 1,500 calories per day. There is no way in the world, even if you ate the perfect diet, that you could ingest all the essential nutrients you need each day when you burn so few calories.

It has been known for years that 24 nutrients are removed from flour during refining. The "enrichment" program returns only 4 nutrients to the refined flour. So 20 out of the 24 nutrients that should be in the flour are still missing. That's an 83% loss. I told this to one of my clients and he was shocked; he thought that enrichment meant that manufacturers *added* nutrients to the ones that were already there— made it better. Dollars and cents rule, not good food for good health.

Avoid white flour and its products, white sugar and its products, and white shortening.

Somehow fat has been identified as the villain, and sugar is off the hook. This is bad science. There is nothing wrong with animal fats: meat fat, butter, and cream. But sugar, my friends, is a killer—avoid it like the plague.

The Food and Nutrition Board, designed to protect our health, is not wholly competent to do so. Today, the FDA, another government watchdog, in place to protect us, does not allow anyone to say that the use of a nutrient or nutritional supplement will protect us, or cure us, of any disease. If one makes statements with health and disease-curing claims for nutrient products, he will be sued. This is in spite of the fact that thousands upon thousands of scientific papers are published in medical and scientific journals proving the efficacy of nutrients in disease prevention and disease elimination.

You can do something about solving the health problem caused by refined foods. There are three choices: 1) eat whole foods, unprocessed and unrefined (if you can find them); 2) encourage food manufacturers to sell whole foods (more of this goes on today than 20 years ago); and 3) use a nutritional supplement with a properly balanced, complete formulation based on the principle of providing all of the essential nutrients.

Environmental Pollution:
Protection by the Use of Nutritional Supplements

Until fairly recently, environmental pollution was rarely considered as a cause of disease. But in 1948, an inversion of air over the steel town of Donora, Pennsylvania, 30 miles north of Pittsburgh, began to change the attitudes of the day.

The high layer of warm air above the four-mile long river valley trapped a deadly mix of sulfur dioxide, carbon monoxide, and metal dust between the hills that straddle the river. The smog was so thick that the fans in the grandstand, watching the high school football team, could not see the players on the field.

By Saturday night, just 24 hours after the disaster began, 11 people were dead, choked to death by the noxious cloud. Nine more died within several hours, and by Monday 7,000 people, more than half the town's population, were ill at home or in hospitals, sickened by the lethal mix.

The Donora tragedy was the first time that public officials recognized the link between air pollution and public health. Later, in 1970, the US Government formed the EPA (Environmental Protection Agency). Its goal was to protect the public from pollution.

Two questions need answers: 1) has the EPA succeeded? 2) Can you trust the Government to protect your health?

In 1975, Dr. Henry Schroeder wrote in his classic book <u>The Poisons Around Us</u> that "the five toxic trace metals—cadmium, beryllium, antimony, mercury, and lead—are extremely important to the health of the public, being involved in half the deaths in the US and much of the disabling diseases."

He was one of the leading scientists involved with establishing standards for clean air. The final limits that were accepted by the committee appalled him. He stated, "These limits are unsafe, and show the abysmal ignorance of the men who proposed them. No, we must do better than that. We will have to rename the Clean Air Act the Dirty Air Act."

Writing about cadmium, a very toxic heavy metal, he states, "It looks innocuous but it has vast potential to poison. It acts subtly and undercover, mimicking diseases in man for which other causes have been proposed, accumulating in the body slowly until the threshold of resistance is overcome, then striking. This subtle property was not recognized until recently. Cadmium is so ubiquitous in our civilization that it is difficult to avoid it."

So, what has happened since 1975 to improve the situation: not much, in spite of all the claims to the contrary.

Cadmium is, still, everywhere in the environment. The pathway it follows into your body is primarily from food, particularly leafy vegetables, grains, and cereals. (What a surprise for all the healthy food eaters!) The tobacco leaf contains substantial amounts of cadmium so that cadmium uptake is virtually doubled in a one-pack-a-day smoker. Cadmium accumulates in the liver and kidneys. It has a long half-life; this means that if you stopped consuming cadmium today (impossible), it would take 17 years for your body to eliminate one-half of the total amount that is now stored in your organs and tissues.

Cadmium interacts with three nutrients essential to human health: calcium, zinc, and iron. It displaces these essential nutrients, literally kicking them out of critical metabolic processes. For example, cadmium inhibits calcium absorption from the intestinal tract. It replaces calcium in bone as does lead, another nasty and highly toxic heavy metal. Osteoporosis is the result.

Recent research shows that there are large amounts of pollution invading our bodies each day. But, a battle rages between groups who proffer opposing viewpoints. On one side are the corporate fat cats and their teams of PhDs, and on the other side are the environmentalists who argue against the growth-at-all-costs attitude of big business.

I tend to support the environmentalists. I think you must seek all methods to protect yourself against the ever-growing menace of toxins and their insidious and destructive pillaging of our health.

Here are some facts from 1998. The evidence is right in front of us. This article appeared in an October issue of the Philadelphia Inquirer, Philadelphia's large daily newspaper. The headline read, **Study: PCBs still in Delaware**. The story states that "despite state efforts to clean up sewage effluent entering the Delaware River, environmental officials were surprised recently to discover that a high concentration of polychlorinated biphenyls in the estuary section of the river are still coming from area treatment plants."

PCBs are human carcinogens. They were "banned" in the 1970's. But, as you can see, they're still around. They can lead to menacing rashes and liver and neurological damage. PCBs are a persistent environmental chemical toxin. Recent work implicates PCB's in many human ills, including the frightful increase in infertility.

Then, just days later, in the same newspaper, the headline read, **Mercury in wells a growing concern**. In this article, the writer presented the saga of a woman suffering from fainting spells, pains and swelling in her arms and legs, and memory loss. Her problems were tied to the pollution of a major aquifer supplying large parts of South Jersey with water.

The water supply of South Jersey has a long history of contamination problems. *The EPA has stated that the water quality in private wells is solely the responsibility of the homeowner* (emphasis added). Another study, conducted by the United States Geological Survey last year, found that 32 of the 34 locations tested had unsafe levels of mercury. And, the state knew as early as 1991 that there were elevated levels of mercury in private wells.

Then, in the same major metropolitan newspaper, on October 25, 1998 (all three articles within 30 days of one another), the headline read, **Radium in N.J. water worse than before**. New Jersey Department of Environmental Protection officials estimate that 75 to 100 public (note public in this report, not private as in the mercury report) water supplies in South Jersey probably will be found unsafe by federal standards due to excess levels of radium. Radium is known to cause bone cancer and poses a special danger for children.

Levels of radium are 160% greater than was known. "There is a risk present in the drinking water that we didn't know was there," said David Huber, head of radiological services of the US EPA in Washington. The radium was found in the Kirkwood-Cohansey Aquifer, a 17-trillion gallon water supply that serves at least 1.2 million people in South Jersey.

Currently there are 100,000 chemicals in commercial use throughout the world and 25,000 of them are known to be hazardous. Recent studies show that 95-100% of people had residues of these chemicals in their body fat!

EPA: National Adipose Tissue Survey

Compound	Sources	% Observation
Styrene	disposable cups, carpet backing	100%
1,4-dichlorobenzene	mothballs, house deodorizers	100%
O C D D (dioxin)	herbicides, auto exhaust	100%
H x C D D (dioxin)	wood treatment, herbicides	98%
Xylene	gasoline, paints	100%
Benzene	gasoline	96%

Table 2. The EPA completed an analysis of human fat samples to determine the level of chemical toxicity contained within the human body. The chart shows the percent of people whose fat samples contained the chemical pollutant listed. Today, samples of human body fat contain residues of from 200-500 different chemical toxins.

The toxic chemical concentration in human fat begs an answer to an important question: What is the threshold level at which these toxins begin to damage your body? Toxicology experts consider cancer the end point of toxic exposure. Usually, to contract cancer, one must be exposed to rather high levels of toxic elements. But, many toxins can damage your body at very low doses of exposure.

This is a very important idea *you must grasp*: most medical and scientific experts do not consider a potential toxin toxic until a diagnosis of cancer is the result. But, today's more enlightened toxicologists recognize that low-levels of toxic agents can begin to do their damage in very subtle ways. This means that cancer is no longer the threshold point of determining damage; a chronic sinusitis or a continually appearing and disappearing skin rash is an example of ways in which the body must deal with the very prevalent effect of a toxic environment.

Compounding this issue is the fact that no one has any idea about the effect of exposure to multiple toxins. The body reacts to these toxins and tries to eliminate them through the kidneys, liver, lungs, skin, mucous membranes, and sweat. Failure to eliminate the full dose leads to a bio-accumulation of the toxins into body organs and systems, particularly body fat.

Many of the reactions that we call colds—including sneezing, coughing, fever, diarrhea, mucous and sinus/lung problems—can, in fact, arise from the body's natural cleansing efforts. Often, these symptoms of cleansing are diagnosed as a bacterial infection or some other type of "disease" and treated with medicines. These medicines cannot be effective because they do not treat the cause of the symptoms and only add a further burden of toxic waste to the body.

An understanding of these issues is of paramount importance to health. Proper diet, in conjunction with an aggressive, well-designed nutritional supplementation program, forms the framework for preventative action against the growing level of pollution.

You cannot count on anyone else, including the government, to protect your health.

The vast majority of medical workers and scientists are wholly unaware of the pervasiveness of the pollution problem and its effects on your health. The recent research now implicates low-dose exposure as a serious threat to our health. Also, the combination of multiple toxins is thoroughly unexplored.

For example, years ago the toxic or unsafe level of lead in the blood was set at 25 micrograms per deciliter. Over the years, as research accumulated, the EPA reduced the toxic level to 10 micrograms per deciliter. Now, more recent research, conducted in the early 1990's, suggests that lead levels as low as 1 microgram per deciliter may cause brain and nerve damage. The average lead level in US citizens is 3 micrograms per deciliter. The government's "safe" level remains at 10 micrograms per deciliter.

Good nutrition, with aggressive nutritional supplementation, can help protect against this toxic overload.

The body has a very sophisticated trash disposal system. The liver is the primary organ in the body for pollutant and toxin elimination. It has a very well developed cadre of about thirty different enzymes which process the thousands of toxins produced each day by our metabolic processes. In addition, these enzymes can process the many chemicals entering our bodies each day through food, air, and water.

One of the most important enzymes in the liver, situated in a strategic position to eliminate pollutants and toxins, is cytochrome P450. This enzyme initiates the first step in the process of preparing an unwanted body toxin for elimination. Nutritional research has identified many nutrients essential to the optimal functioning of this enzyme. The table outlines several key nutrients required by the body to maximally manufacture cytochrome P450. Deficiencies of these nutrients compromise the manufacture of the enzyme.

Dietary Changes	Effect
Mineral deficiencies	↓
Calcium	↓
Copper	↓
Iron	↓
Magnesium	↓
Zinc	↓
Vitamin deficiencies	
Vitamin C	↓
Vitamin E	↓
B complex	↓
Protein deficiencies	↓
Starvation (more than 2 days)	↓

↓ = decreasing ability to remove toxins

Table 3.

In summary, we are exposed to attack by many foreign and toxic elements in our environment. Optimum nutrition is extremely important in charging our body's internal cleansing system with the ability to flush away these damaging agents. Unfortunately, our modern diet will not meet the need: this is without a doubt; all of the nutritional surveys over the last thirty years continually show that we are deficient in many key nutrients.

In spite of what you hear, we are not adequately nourished. Further, the environment is more hostile each day. Government officials and industry leaders proclaim at the top of their voices, "The air is clean, the water is clean, our diets are pure and wholesome." Nonsense. It just isn't so.

Take charge of your own health. You are solely responsible to protect your health and the health of your family. High quality nutritional supplements, including all the essential nutrients in the proper balance with high absorption and assimilation properties, are insurance you cannot afford to pass up.

chapter 4

Nutritional Basics

In Dr. Roger Williams' classic book <u>Nutrition Against Disease</u>, he describes the reasons why the medical profession is so opposed to the idea that there is a relationship between nutrition and disease. He tells the story about the resistance experienced by Louis Pasteur from the medical men of his day against his theory that microbes (bacteria) caused disease. As is often the case, the next generation of doctors, however, accepted Pasteur's theory of the microbial origin of disease; they embraced it.

In fact, they carried the idea even further than Pasteur would have by insisting that all diseases are microbial in origin. These ideas became so entrenched in the medical way of thinking that many doctors, in subsequent years, continued to resist the idea that a nutritional deficiency might, in any way, impact upon health. When Dr. Casimir Funk set forth in 1911 the "vitamin hypothesis," suggesting that several major diseases were nutritional in origin, his ideas were rejected at first and then, grudgingly, accepted later on. This series of historical facts has tended to turn medical thinking *away from*, rather than *toward*, nutrition.

Dr. Williams describes what he refers to as the ***Nutritional Chain of Life***. He states that nourishing food must be a complex mixture of chemicals in about the right proportions. Included in this food must be about 10 or more amino acids, about 15 vitamins, and 15 minerals, all in addition to the fuel we need each day from carbohydrates, fats, and proteins, to power our bodies.

Dr. Williams predicted, in 1971, that in the near future, people would have a vastly increased interest in the *internal environment* (of the body), paralleling the surge of national and worldwide interest in the *external environment* (the land, water, and air) that he was observing at that time when his book was published.

I have already described the dangers implicit in the external environment today. So imagine, as difficult as it is to protect the external environment, against all the in-fighting among the various vested interests, it is that much more difficult to protect our internal environment, and for one simple reason: we can't see it! Very few people even consider what is going on inside their body because they cannot visualize it.

Over time, our body begins to slowly break down because of the onslaught of both environmental pollutants and poor nutritional habits, similar to the way a speck of rust gradually begins to erode the metal structure of a pipe. Unfortunately, because we cannot see it, our awareness of this damage occurs so late that only the physician, with his interior-observing tests, is able to diagnose our deterioration. Then, it is often too late.

To protect our health, we must prevent illness. Prevention is the key, and one of the hallmarks of prevention is good nutrition. Our body needs, absolutely needs, a specific amount of nutrients each day to remain healthy. If your diet is low in one, or more than one nutrient then, over time, a nutritional deficiency may arise. If the nutrient intake is too low, the end result may be sickness or even death.

This was the purpose of the nutrition studies during the first half of the nineteenth century: to discover the purpose and function of the chemicals that foods contained and how they affected our health. But today, the emphasis has switched to the concept of Optimal Nutrition. That's why there is such an interest in designer foods and nutritional supplements.

To sustain life the body needs 1) air, 2) water, 3) food fuel as a source of energy, and 4) maintenance chemicals: a whole gamut of biochemicals that we need to supply to our cells so that their metabolic machinery can function optimally.

Energy is the number one requirement of the body (air and water are absolutely required as well). Without an adequate supply of energy, we waste away and die. Protein, fats, and carbohydrates are the energy macronutrients that make up food. And there are endless arguments about the importance of each of these three macronutrients to health. A discussion of this topic is beyond the scope of this treatise.

The current research emphasis today focuses on the maintenance chemicals.

Today, however, most people do not suffer from outright nutrient deficiencies.

Essential Nutrients

I have developed, here, the idea of the importance of good nutrition and described the difficulty of receiving good nutrition solely from our food intake. I will, now, begin to describe the elements required to provide your body with all of the essential nutrients through an appropriate nutritional supplementation program.

RDI (Reference Daily Intake) and RDA (Recommended Dietary Allowance)

Vitamins and minerals are essential to good health and even to life itself. But how do we know whether we're getting sufficient nutrients to insure our well being? For approximately 50 years, the Recommended Daily Allowances (RDAs) were our guidelines. They were the United States Food and Nutrition Board's estimates of the amount of nutrients required by most people to prevent deficiency symptoms.

RDAs served as a framework for the medical community's opinion that supplementation was unnecessary. Statements, such as "We can get everything we need from a well-balanced diet" and "Vitamin and mineral supplements are a waste of money," are based on wide-spread acceptance of these guidelines, above.

One of the primary functions of the RDAs was to provide individuals with information about their essential nutrient intake. Scientists evaluated the data from various research studies over the years and set the criteria accordingly. In setting the amount they considered to be adequate, they added a fudge-factor: a small percent increase over the basic amount adequate to provide good health. The purpose of this so-called fudge-factor was to take into account variations in lifestyle.

After their development, the RDAs were periodically evaluated and updated, based on a continuing analysis of our rapidly expanding knowledge of nutrition. But in 1985, when the new guidelines were targeted for release, there was such widespread disagreement among the scientists involved in setting the new standards that the National Research Council was unable to issue the scheduled release until 1989.

Reams of scientific experiments had been reported over the years suggesting that higher intakes of essential nutrients would help improve health. This led to significant disagreement among scientists, including nutritionists, physicians, and researchers.

In 1993, the Nutrition Labeling and Education Act replaced the RDAs with the RDIs (Reference Daily Intake). Since January 1997, the RDA nomenclature has no longer been used. However, just like the RDAs, the RDIs have three basic problems:

1) One cannot get all of the nutrients one needs from today's food,

2) RDIs only reflect amounts that are adequate to prevent nutrient-deficiency diseases and are not tailored for individual needs,

3) RDIs do not address or consider *optimum health* or the prevention of degenerative diseases such as cancer and heart disease.

The notion that one can achieve an adequate dietary intake of essential nutrients from food has proven false. Unfortunately, medical doctors, who provide dietary recommendations to their patients, are the most vocal group perpetuating the idea that our dietary intake is adequate to meet our daily nutritional needs. On this subject, one should not listen to the advice of medical doctors, whose training in nutritional science is non-existent, because they steadfastly continue to operate under the myth that a well-balanced diet can meet our nutritional needs.

It is virtually impossible for physicians to keep abreast of the overwhelming amount of nutritional information published each year. Even if they could keep abreast, they were not trained in nutrition basics or in nutrition science and, for many of them, it is like reading a foreign language. Nutrition education is woefully lacking in medical schools throughout the United States.

Today, it is almost impossible to ingest all the essential nutrients that we need each day for optimal health. There are two primary impediments: first, many of our foods are depleted nutritionally; the nutrient content of the soil on which our foods are grown is significantly lower than it was at the turn of the century. Food processing also depletes food of essential nutrients. I've already discussed this in detail as it relates, in particular, to sugar and flour products.

An additional impediment to ingesting all the essential nutrients every day is that Americans are so physically inactive that we require fewer calories each day to meet our energy output. We have experienced a large decrease in energy requirements since the time of our ancestors, just 70-90 years ago. Several well-respected researchers have claimed that we need to eat at least 2,500 calories per day to attain an adequate intake of essential vitamins and minerals. This calculation also assumes that the food that we supply to our body is unprocessed and nutritionally complete. Food storage requirements today make it difficult to achieve this goal.

For example, the vitamin C content of apples may fall by 2/3 after only two or three months. Potatoes may have 30 mg of vitamin C per 100 grams when they're freshly harvested in the fall, but by spring-time they may have only 8 mg per 100 grams. By summer, they have practically none. Green vegetables suffer even more: they lose almost all their vitamin C after a few days of being stored at room temperature. Everyone knows that orange juice is high in vitamin C, but few people realize that an orange loses 30 percent of its vitamin C after it is squeezed. The processing of oranges into non-fortified commercial juice obliterates the natural vitamin C content.

The heat, light, water, and chemicals used to process foods further deplete their nutrients. Blanching, a process that vegetables undergo before they're canned or frozen, can destroy up to 60% of the vitamin C content, 40% of the riboflavin, and 30% of the thiamin. The sterilization process used to can foods further destroys vitamins. For example, about 39% of the vitamin A is destroyed and 69% of the thiamin during the canning process.

Today, the average calorie consumption for women between ages 19 to 50 is approximately 1,500-1,700 calories per day. Even at that level of calorie intake, the nation is becoming fatter by the year. This is primarily a function of our lower level of physical activity. Labor saving devices have made it very difficult for people to exert the amount of energy each day that they need to exert in order to maintain their proper body weight, even with three heart-pounding aerobic sessions per week.

The RDIs are a "one-size-fits-all" recommendation. They were designed to satisfy the need of the mythical "average healthy person," not to meet the specific needs of an individual. They are a group average. In addition to the individual biological blueprint each of us comes into the world with, we continue to change throughout life. We have different experiences and exposures to damaging agents such as pollution, stress, disease, drug therapy, and aging. Our changing experiences and exposures increase our need for specific nutrients. They can interfere with nutrient metabolism and affect our nutritional needs.

The RDAs and RDIs were established as guidelines for preventing overt symptoms of vitamin and mineral deficiencies leading to specific diseases. The guidelines were not designed to address the question of the necessary nutrient intake we need to achieve optimal health. The scientists and medical professionals who were a part of these advisory panels were trained to believe that nutrition played a small role in human health. They never even considered that an increased nutritional intake of higher amounts or larger quantities of specific nutrients could affect health in a positive way.

Recently, scientific efforts have moved us away from the nutrition research of the mid-century, which concerned itself solely with the idea of nutritional deficiencies. Science, today, views nutritional supplementation as a way to optimize health. State-of-the-art biochemical techniques show that the classic, overt vitamin deficiency diseases, such as beri-beri and pellagra, are merely the last event in a long chain-of-reactions, similar to the way an erupting volcano or earthquake is the last dramatic step in a series of underground processes.

When we do not get enough of a specific vitamin or mineral, the initial reactions occur on the molecular level. The first event that happens is a depletion of the vitamin and mineral stores in the body's reserve storage areas, followed by a reduction of the essential nutrient in the cell matrix itself. This, in turn, brings about changes at the cellular level. The cells of the body—which depend upon millions of intracellular enzymes to process the broken down food chemicals to energy and for the synthesis of new cellular materials—can no longer carry out their normal functions.

When nutrient depletion is prolonged and severe, the classic, clinical signs of nutritional deficiency appear, including disease. Disruption of optimal cellular function, however, always precedes the appearance of classic deficiency disease.

These cellular changes, degrading (on a continuum) from optimal function towards disease, are known as *sub-clinical deficiencies*. They are not the kind of deficiencies that your doctor would necessarily discover through his or her routine physical exam and blood testing. But while they may not be obvious, easily definable, or immediately debilitating, these deficiencies do have an affect on the body's well-being.

The subtle, sub-clinical changes, due to poor or even marginally poor nutrition, may be responsible for a broad range of non-specific conditions that can, at first, be merely annoying but gradually increase in impact, reducing our overall health and quality of life. These conditions can include chronic fatigue, skin problems, recurrent or lingering infections or colds, digestive problems, sleep problems, headaches, or hormonal problems, depression, and nervousness. Poor nutrient intake may also leave us more vulnerable to genetically predisposed diseases such as cardiovascular disease, diabetes, and cancer.

In the past, the medical community has been very skeptical about the use of nutritional supplements. However, today's younger physicians, because of the onslaught of scientific research supporting nutritional supplement use, are encouraging their patients to use a nutritional supplementation program.

Since many people are interested in attaining a state of optimum health while preventing disease, we must ingest each day the optimum—not minimum—amounts of vitamins and minerals. The need for *optimum daily intake* is based on five factors:

1. The RDIs are generally based on an amount that simply prevents classic deficiency diseases.

2. The RDIs do not take into account preventative or therapeutic levels of nutrients.

3. Because of many factors, including loss of nutrients from shipping, storage, and processing, the foods available to us do not contain the amounts of vitamins and minerals they should contain.

4. Owing to the constant bombardment of stress factors, from pollution to emotional stress, we require higher levels of vitamins and minerals than originally thought.

5. The vitamins and minerals in foods and supplements are never 100% absorbed.

Reading the RDIs on a Nutritional Supplement Label

Labeling laws established by the Food and Drug Administration (FDA) require manufacturers to list the RDIs (RDIs are replacing RDAs) for all nutrients contained within a nutritional supplement. Consumers can learn a lot about the nutritional supplement they choose by understanding how to read the label.

Now, we have established that the RDIs are inadequate to meet your nutrient needs. Nonetheless, do not totally discard the information the RDIs provide as if it were useless—it is not. Use the RDIs as a starting point. Therefore, your first action is to check to see if the nutritional supplement that you have selected contains at least 100% of the RDI for each nutrient listed. Your second action is to make sure that the nutritional supplement that you have selected contains all the essential nutrients and that they are in the correct balance.

Table 4 at the end of this section defines the essential daily nutrient needs in a basic vitamin and mineral supplement to provide "insurance" against nutrient deficiency (take a few minutes to review Table 4 now). The ranges presented are from the opinions of various international experts. These values reflect my own opinion as well. Remember, the goal of a nutritional supplement is not to meet all of your daily needs because you will consume many of the essential nutrients from your daily diet: the goal of the supplement is just that: to supplement your daily intake of essential nutrients from food.

Typically, what you will discover is that most nutritional supplements in the marketplace provide you with a *megadose* of some nutrients and a *deficiency* of many other nutrients. The most common formulation error is that the manufacturer will load up on the inexpensive B vitamin family nutrients, such as thiamin, riboflavin, and niacin and scrimp on the more expensive, bulky materials such as the minerals.

However, minerals are far more important than vitamins as a first choice in a nutritional supplement. For example, looking at a supplement label for vitamin B1 (thiamin), you'll very often discover that the amount of the vitamin in the supplement is significantly higher than the RDI. Often the amount in the formulation is anywhere from 500% to 5,000% higher than the RDI.

Now, I don't agree with the RDIs; I do believe that they are too low. However, a great deal of scientific research went into establishing the RDI values, and I don't believe we should throw the baby out with the bath water and simply discard fifty years of research into the nutritional requirements of humans.

Although I do agree that the amounts are too low, the important question becomes, "How much higher should they be?" This is a very important question to ask, and, in my experience, it is not asked or answered by many manufacturers. Their attitude is that the RDIs are too low and that the Food and Nutrition Board is a conservative bunch of no-brained, closed-minded scientists. So, instead of using the existing, voluminous base of scientific data as a starting point, they yell and scream to scrap it altogether, ascribing no value whatsoever to the fundamental research that has gone on for many years.

I believe this research serves as a sound base. And, starting from that position, we can now frame the appropriate questions. The first question is how much should we increase the nutrient level in the supplements that we choose? And the second question is which nutrients should we adjust and which ones should we leave alone?

Most manufacturers megadose the B vitamins. And buyers seem to become really excited by this. I think we all suffer from the "more-is-better" syndrome. But, to formulate an optimal amount and ration of nutrients, it is not necessary to increase the quantity of a nutrient 100 or 1,000 percent over the recommended RDI for one to attain the optimal intake of a certain nutrient.

Certainly, in the class of the B vitamins, five times the RDI, or as much as 10 times the RDI, is adequate. Research supports this. But for some of the other nutrients, particularly the minerals, increases above and beyond the RDI should be very carefully considered for each individual mineral and for the ratio of one mineral to the other.

Later in this monograph, you'll read about interactions between various vitamins and minerals and also about mineral to mineral interactions. You'll discover that there are some very significant dangers implicit in increasing the amounts of a nutrient that you ingest and also in disrupting the delicate proportions and balance between individual nutrients with one another.

Vitamins A, D, and E are also essential nutrients and considered as the **First Line of Defense** against free radical damage in the body. These vitamins are considered as the major antioxidants within the body. But, we also have to be careful about how many antioxidants we ingest each day. Recent research into antioxidant use has demonstrated that too many antioxidants can damage our immune system and alter the function in a negative way for our organs and systems. I discuss the results of these studies more fully in a later section about antioxidants.

In summary, use the label information to guide you about the adequacy of the nutritional formulation that you have selected. The product should be well balanced, adequate in nutrient content, and the *chemical sources* for the various nutrients should be the best you can buy (I will discuss later this all-important issue of the chemical sources of nutrients). **Look to minerals first and then vitamins second.**

Nutrient	Lower Range	Upper Range
Vitamin A (acetate)	2,500 IU	25,000 IU
Vitamin A (from beta carotene)	5,000 IU	25,000 IU
Vitamin C	100 mg	3,000 mg
Vitamin D	100 IU	400 IU
Vitamin E	40 IU	800 IU
Vitamin K	60 mcg	300 mcg
Vitamin B1 (thiamine)	2 mg	100 mg
Vitamin B2 (riboflavin)	2 mg	50 mg
Vitamin B3 (niacin)	20 mg	500 mg
Vitamin B6 (pyridoxine)	3 mg	100 mg
Vitamin B12	9 mcg	400 mcg
Pantothenic Acid	15 mg	100 mg
Biotin	100 mcg	300 mcg
Folic Acid	400 mcg	800 mcg
Choline	10 mg	100 mg
Inositol	10 mg	100 mg
Minerals		
Calcium*	250 mg	1,000 mg
Magnesium*	200 mg	500 mg
Iron*	15 mg	30 mg
Zinc*	15 mg	40 mg
Copper*	2 mg	5 mg
Manganese*	5 mg	15 mg
Chromium*	200 mcg	400 mcg
Selenium*	50 mcg	200 mcg
Boron*	1 mg	6 mg
Molybdenum*	2 mcg	25 mcg

* Daily intake is dependent on the chemical source of for the nutrient: amino acid chelate absorption rate is 200-300% higher than milk or other sources: so less is more.

Table 4.

chapter 5

A Must for Understanding Mineral Nutrition: What Are Elemental Levels of Minerals

Are you really getting what the label says? This may surprise you, but most often the tablet or capsule does not contain what you think you are getting. Minerals come as a complex of two or more chemicals: 1) the mineral itself, which is called the *elemental mineral* and 2) the *chemical source* of the elemental mineral. An example is calcium carbonate in which the *elemental* mineral is calcium and the *chemical source* of the elemental calcium is calcium carbonate. Others include magnesium oxide (the *elemental* mineral is magnesium and the *chemical source* is magnesium oxide) and ferrous fumarate (the *elemental* mineral is ferrous—that's iron—and the *chemical source* is ferrous fumarate).

Why is this important? Let's use the example of calcium carbonate. Everyone knows that an adequate intake of calcium is important to health. Many people use a calcium supplement to make-up for the shortfall created by a too low dietary intake from food sources. Looking at the supplement label, we see that it claims:

3 tablets per days provide: Calcium 1,000 mg

The source of the calcium listed on the label is calcium carbonate. Calcium is bound chemically to carbonate in a 1:1 ratio. This means that for every calcium molecule there is one molecule of carbonate. Next, we must figure exactly how much elemental calcium is in the molecule of calcium carbonate so we know exactly how much calcium we are ingesting. To do this, we must know the molecular weight of the individual chemicals. The following charts provide the molecular weights of some common minerals and the chemicals they are combined with.

Mineral Molecular Weight

Mineral	Molecular Weight
Magnesium	24.31
Calcium	40.08
Zinc	65.38
Copper	63.55
Iron	55.85
Manganese	54.94
Chromium	51.96

Table 5.

Molecular Weight of Chemicals Bound to Minerals

Chemical	Molecular Weight
Citrate	192.12
Carbonate	60.00
Gluconate	196.16
Oxide	16.00
Glycinate	75.07
Lactate	90.08
Sulfate	98.08
Fumarate	114.06

Table 6.

Mineral Compounds: Their Weights & Elemental Mineral Content

Chemical Compound	Molecular Ratios	% Elemental Mineral
Calcium Citrate	Calcium:Citrate (3:2)	24.1
Ferrous Fumarate	Ferrous: Fumarate (1:1)	32.9
Calcium Carbonate	Calcium:Carbonate (1:1)	40.4
Magnesium Citrate	Magnesium:Citrate (2:3)	16.2
Calcium Glycinate	Calcium:Glycine (1:2)	20.0
Calcium Gluconate	Calcium:Gluconate (2:1)	9.3
Zinc Phosphate	Zinc:Phosphate (3:2)	50.8
Zinc Picolinate	Zinc:Picolinate (1:2)	21.0

Table 7.

Using the tables above, we see that 1,000 milligrams (mg) of calcium carbonate yield only 400 mg of elemental calcium. The Reference Daily Intake (RDI) for calcium is 1,000 mg. At 1,000 mg, as the label states, you are ingesting 100% of your needed amount. But, since 60% of the compound is carbonate, and not calcium, you are ingesting only 40% of your RDI for calcium. This is a long way from what you need each day.

To reach your RDI, you would need to actually take 6 1/2 tablets or capsules each day instead of the 3 that were recommended! And that's just for calcium. Imagine for a moment that you have purchased a daily multivitamin and mineral supplement that promises to deliver the ideal amount and proportions of your daily nutrient needs for all 30 essential vitamins and minerals in 3 to 6 tablets or capsules per day.

I've already outlined the approximately 40 essential nutrients (10 of which are amino acids, leaving about 30 nutrients that are vitamins and minerals) that you need each day. How can a manufacturer possibly get that much stuff into just 3 to 6 tablets or capsules per day to meet your needs? The answer is that they can't; it's impossible.

Let's put some numbers to it. A typical double zero (00) capsule holds about 1,100 mg of nutrient powder. This will vary because some nutrients are more dense (weigh more per unit volume) than other nutrients; therefore they take up less space in the capsule, allowing more milligrams of ingredients to fit inside the capsule. The actual size of this capsule is approximately:

Let's look at an example: our goal is to have a supplement deliver, in capsule form, a daily requirement for three minerals: calcium, magnesium, and zinc. The following table provides the sources for the nutrients and the milligrams of elemental mineral and its chemical source.

Source	% Elemental	Daily Goal (mg)	Amount of Chemical Source Required (mg)
Calcium Citrate	24	800	3,333
Magnesium Citrate	16	400	2,500
Zinc Picolinate	21	15	70.5
		Total mg needed	5,904

Table 7.

The data in the table show that to meet your daily needs for just three essential mineral nutrients, the capsules must contain 5,904 mg of source chemical. These three nutrients alone would require 5.4 capsules just to hold this much material.

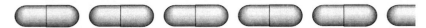

Many people have heard of Centrum®. It is a multivitamin mineral tablet. Each tablet weighs about 1,500 mg and is stated to provide you with your one-a-day nutrient requirements. It would take almost 4 Centrum® tablets to hold just the three nutrients listed in the table above.

The important point is that many companies <u>claim</u> that their product has the <u>potency</u> required to meet your daily need. Now, you don't have to study the tables above very long to understand that this is impossible. It takes a <u>specific quantity</u> of a nutrient supplement to meet your daily needs. *You simply cannot get around this.* The nutrient weighs something and takes up a specific volume of space. It cannot be compressed to any large degree so that it takes up less space. It just is and that's that.

This same scenario exists for all nutrients, but especially for minerals. <u>To know how much of a mineral you receive each day, you must know the source of the mineral</u>. There are more than 500 sources for minerals used in the supplement market.

Many people look for a supplement whose directions and marketing message claim that only 1 capsule per day, or 3 per day, or 6 per day will cover their nutrient needs. People can't or don't like to swallow pills. The fewer they have to swallow each day, the happier they are. But, if you want your supplement to provide what you need, then forget about 1 pill per day.

If you believe you can do it in one pill per day, you are suffering from wishful thinking. Forget the wishes; open up your mouth, pour in a lot of water, and swallow. Do yourself a favor and take what you need. The one-pill-meets-your-needs salesman is selling you a bill-of-goods, and he's emptying your wallet by scamming you. I cannot stress this enough: if you want a product that will meet your daily needs for <u>all</u> of the essential nutrients, then it must take up space, and it requires a significant number of capsules to do the job. Nothing less will do, and nothing less is worth your money.

chapter 6

Nutrient Absorption

How Much of the Elemental Nutrient Enters Into Your Blood and Then Into Your Body's Cells

Minerals

As important as ingesting the right amount of nutrients is, there is another concern that is even more important. That is: how much of the nutrient crosses the intestinal cells and travels into the blood so that it can be delivered to the cells of all the systems and organs in the body.

Absorption is the process by which the body "takes in" a substance. A substance can be beneficial or deleterious to the body. Minerals are metals, and metals can benefit or harm. Examples of metals that cause harm are lead (this is a well-known heavy metal toxin that is highly prevalent in the environment) and cadmium (this is another heavy metal toxin that is present in the environment). In fact, the most significant sources of cadmium in the environment today are grains, fruits, and vegetables. The reason for this is the content of cadmium in pesticides and insecticides.

Absorption is a complex and highly developed process. The skin, lungs, and gastrointestinal tract (GI) are the main barriers separating the inside of your body from the outside environment. It is important to realize that your whole GI tract is, anatomically, considered to be *outside* of your body. Therefore, a nutrient must be permitted to enter *into* your body by a passageway through the protective barrier of the GI tract.

This is the process of absorption. The quantity of nutrients absorbed depends on the chemical composition of the nutrient. This determines how easily the nutrient can cross the protective barrier that prevents the entry of foreign matter *into* your body.

The chemical composition of the nutrient also determines how it will interact with foods and nutrients contained in the digestive tract. These nutrients compete against one another for passage across the protective barrier of intestinal cells.

Modern science is, just now, beginning to explore the differences existing between various nutrient complexes and their rates of absorption. Once absorbed, the nutrient distributes itself, via the blood, to different body organs and systems. The cells of the organs or systems act as another barrier to the entry of a nutrient into the cell itself. Once the nutrient enters the cell, the cellular metabolic machinery can construct new chemicals from it to do the work of the cell.

You can see from the above scenario that there are many impediments to a nutrient reaching the site where it will be used. Therefore, absorption represents one of the most important considerations in nutrient selection. For example, the iron in spinach is very poorly absorbed from the gut whereas the iron in meat is absorbed 15 times more.

The chemical composition of the raw materials making up nutritional supplements is of paramount importance. This concept is little discussed and poorly understood by most purchasers of products. It is also poorly understood by most supplement manufactures. *Their most important concern is the final selling price of the product and the net, bottom-line profit they will realize.*

Absorption of Calcium

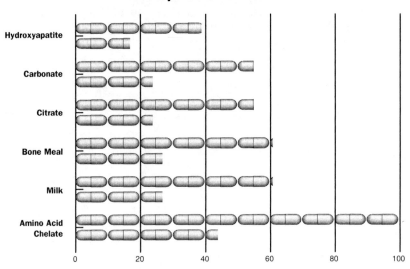

Graph 3. The chemical source of a nutrient is critical in the absorption process from the gastrointestinal tract. In this graph, the amino acid chelate form of calcium is compared with other chemical sources of calcium. The absorption from the intestine of elemental calcium from the amino acid chelate is 44% and serves as the basis of comparison for the other calcium sources.

For example, the gastrointestinal absorption of calcium from milk is about 27%, but compared with the amino acid chelate, calcium absorption from milk is only 61% of that realized from the chelate source. Calcium citrate, hydroxyapatite, and bone meal are popular sources as supplements for calcium. They are poor sources compared with the amino acid chelate. Calcium carbonate is the most common chemical source for calcium supplementation, but pales in comparison to the chelate form. Regular use of calcium carbonate can cause Milk Alkali Syndrome which may lead to poor absorption of the all-important proteins in your diet and, if continued long enough and in a high enough dose, may lead to kidney damage and failure.

Diet composition is a major factor determining the absorption of nutrients from the intestinal tract. Our modern day emphasis on high fiber intake is having a deleterious affect on nutrient absorption. This is particularly important in mineral nutrition, and I've emphasized that mineral supplementation is more important than vitamin supplementation.

Any factor that decreases mineral absorption will affect the health of the body. In 1942, Drs. McCance and Widdowson observed losses of both calcium and magnesium in humans fed whole wheat bread. Later, Dr. Prasad demonstrated evidence of zinc deficiency in humans fed larger amounts of dietary fiber.

Several minerals of major importance to human health are divalent cations. Whoa, what's this all about? "Divalent cation" is chemical jargon that says the mineral has two electrical charges. The key minerals with two charges are calcium, zinc, iron, and magnesium. All this means to you is that the chemistry of some fibers allows them to react with the essential minerals, binding them up so tightly that the minerals cannot be absorbed from the intestine and, as a result, pass out of the body without being absorbed.

One of the most popular fibers sold in stores nationwide today is manufactured from the husk of psyllium seed. In fact, it is the primary ingredient in Metamucil®. Studies with psyllium have shown that it depresses the absorption of magnesium and has some negative effects on the absorption of copper and zinc.

Wheat decreases calcium, magnesium, and phosphorous absorption, and wheat bran decreases iron absorption. With the decreased consumption of red meat, which contains significant amounts of iron in a highly available and absorbable form, inadequate iron nutrition, particularly in women and children, has become a significant health problem.

The chemical source of the nutritional supplement also impacts on the absorption of the multi-nutrients contained within the tablet or capsule. The following tables show the effect of zinc absorption on calcium absorption into the blood. Table 8 shows that the chemical source of the mineral element determines the absorption amount. The amino acid chelate of zinc is absorbed significantly more than other sources.

Table 9 shows that zinc absorption (from zinc sulfate, a poor chemical source of zinc), decreases when the zinc supplement is given at the same time as a calcium supplement.

Mineral Absorption Rates in Milligrams

	Mineral Chelate	Sulfate	Oxide	Carbonate
Zinc Source	191	84	66	87

Table 8.

Ca Carbonate and Ca Citrate on Zinc Absorption

Supplement Source	Plasma Zinc	Zinc Absorption %
Zinc Sulfate alone	1,561.7	100%
Zinc Sulfate with Calcium Carbonate	438.4	28%
Zinc Sulfate with Calcium Citrate	308.0	19.7%

Table 9.

The following chart further demonstrates how important the chemical source of the mineral is to achieve high levels of nutrient absorption. The amino acid chelate absorbs from the intestine 3.7 times more than the ferrous sulfate and ferrous fumarate forms which are the primary and cheapest forms that manufacturers use in mineral formulations. You know the old saying, "You get what you pay for!"

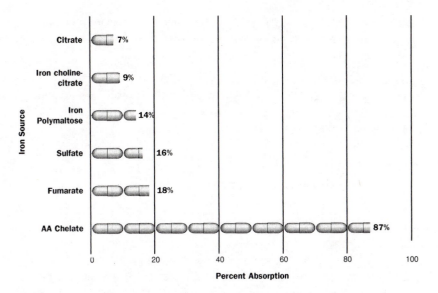

Graph 4.

Let's paint a picture of a day in the life of a nutritional supplement user. He starts the day off with a healthy breakfast of high-fiber cereal and low-fat milk. His multi-vitamin and mineral supplement is advertised to provide his daily requirements for all the essential nutrients. It requires three tablets. The mineral's chemical sources are citrates, gluconates, sulfates, and carbonates.

It appears that he has done everything right. But, unknown to him, a war is about to break out in his stomach. His high-fiber meal binds to the various minerals as they break away from their chemical source. The fiber, rushing helter-skelter through his intestinal tract, carries the essential minerals with it on its way out of the body.

The minerals remaining now try to cross the intestinal cell barriers into the bloodstream where they can travel to the body's organs. Here, another battle rages: the minerals, now separated from their chemical source, actually fight one another for absorption across the cell wall: calcium and zinc fight against iron, copper fights zinc. The vitamin and mineral supplement also contains various herbs that now join the brutal battle, and they also bind up the minerals and other nutrients in a chemical headlock, yielding more non-absorbable nutrient complexes.

I'm sure this comes as a surprise; surely you thought all supplements were the same. Not everything is what it appears to be; you must be very careful in choosing your nutritional supplement.

The herbal supplement revolution is now underway, with major international pharmaceutical companies entering the arena. The chemicals in many of these herbs have a strong binding power for minerals, and they will inhibit the intestinal absorption of these essential nutrients.

Effects of Heavy Metals on Essential Mineral Absorption

Another major issue is the effect of environmental heavy metal toxicity. This fact alone makes nutritional supplementation an absolute necessity. The major toxic metals are lead, cadmium, and mercury. Your body has no nutritional need for these metals, and there may be no tissue concentration at which there is not a toxic effect from having them in your body. Interactions with, or deficiencies of, essential metals such as calcium and magnesium have a role in increasing the severity of the heavy metal's toxic effect.

Lead affects calcium absorption, both from the GI tract and from the blood into the target organ. It also affects nutrient retention in the organ or system. For example, lead actually displaces calcium from bone and leads to osteoporosis. Lead concentration in the intestine decreases calcium absorption. High levels of calcium can protect against lead absorption.

Mercury is another toxic metal that is prevalent in the environment. Most people have mercury in their teeth in the form of amalgam (silver) fillings. Selenium protects against acute mercury toxicity. Selenium works together with vitamin E and other antioxidants to provide this protective effect.

A recent study evaluated multiple chemical sources of calcium for lead content. Remember, lead displaces calcium; it has a stronger electrochemcial attraction for the chemical source that normally, in the absence of lead, combines with calcium. Therefore, it is not unexpected that lead would appear in commercial sources of calcium supplements.

The study showed that all of the products using dolomite or bone meal as a calcium source contained lead levels that were above the safe limit recommended by the government. Only 2 out of 25 of the unrefined calcium carbonate products met the standards required for safety.

Dr. Robert Goyer, however, states that <u>no</u> amount of lead may be safe. So, even if the product meets the standards, so what? Is that good enough?

Again, the safe bet is to use a pure amino acid chelate (see next paragraph for a description of a mineral chelate) because the product is 100% mineral and amino acid. Properly manufactured, using only pure, pharmaceutical grade raw materials that have no contamination, chelated minerals are the best source for mineral supplementation. <u>Stay away from the natural sources of calcium such as bone meal, dolomite, and oyster shells</u>, unless the manufacturer proves that the source is not contaminated. (And even if that is the case, the absorption rates for these chemical sources are much less than the rates for an amino acid chelate).

Amino Acid Chelates

The use of mineral chelates is an absolute requirement for proper nutritional supplement formulations. Amino acid chelates combine the essential mineral with an amino acid. Amino acids are the building blocks for proteins and there are 22 known amino acids. The strong chemical bond between the amino acid and mineral yields a product that does not break down in the stomach. This is critical for the successful absorption of the minerals later on as they move into the intestinal tract where absorption occurs.

Amino acids are highly absorbed; they are absorbed as amino acids and the mineral is "smuggled" across the intestinal cells into the blood disguised as an amino acid. This is why chelated minerals do not compete against other minerals for absorption. Nutritional supplements using 100% mineral chelates provide the highest levels of absorption for essential minerals.

Again, you must be very wary as a label reader. It is relatively inexpensive to provide the minerals needed by the body <u>in low amounts</u> as chelates. Copper requirements are about 2 milligrams per day. That's not much quantity or volume; it won't take up too much space in a capsule. Iron and zinc requirements are about 15 milligrams per day. Again, not too much.

But calcium and magnesium are another story. You need hundreds of milligrams of these nutrients each day. This is expensive and the nutrient takes up a large amount of space in the capsule. Also, since chelates are mostly amino acids and a small amount of mineral, it takes a lot of the raw material to provide your daily requirement of the essential nutrients.

For example, a calcium amino acid chelate is about 14% calcium. So, out of 1,000 milligrams of raw material, only 140 milligrams is calcium. To receive 500 milligrams of elemental calcium, the capsule must contain a total of 3,570 milligrams including both the calcium plus the amino acid that it is chelated to (its source)!

A double 0 (00) capsule (standard size used in nutritional supplements) holds about 1,100 milligrams. If you use a mineral acid chelate, then you need over 3 capsules per day just to meet your calcium need.

Amino acid chelate has become a buzzword in the nutritional supplement industry. Today, more manufacturers use amino acid chelates as one of the chemical sources for the minerals in their nutritional supplements. Most manufacturers, however, only use a pinch of amino acid chelate as a source because of its cost and because of the space that it takes up inside the capsule (which also increases cost).

But, and this is a big but, when they list calcium, for example, on the label, you often see several ingredients listed as the chemical sources for the calcium such as calcium carbonate, di-calcium phosphate, and amino acid chelate. It is most likely however, that the amino acid chelate represents *only a small portion* of the total raw material. That's why it is important that the mineral component of your daily, essential nutritional supplement contains only 100% amino acid chelates.

High levels of absorption require the proper raw materials. The nutrient formulation must also be properly balanced so that you can achieve optimal levels of nutrient supply to your cells. There are many hazardous roads that can block nutrient absorption and use.

Summary of Mineral Absorption

In summary, two major changes have occurred in industrialized countries over the last two decades that may have harmful affects on the health of people. These changes are 1) the increase in fiber intake and 2) the increase in nutritional supplementation by the public. Two surprises! Who would have ever thought that these two actions, that most people believe to be positive, healthy actions, could have a negative health effect?

Why is fiber a problem? A high-fiber intake decreases mineral absorption. This may offset, or counter, any health benefits derived from increased fiber intake. One way around this problem is the use of properly designed nutritional supplements that include the use of the right raw ingredients and the correct proportion of essential nutrients. For example, minerals, as amino acid chelates, are not affected by the fiber content of the diet and their absorption rate remains high in the presence or absence of fiber.

The second major change is that up to 50% of the US population now uses supplements, and this number is increasing every day. Manufacturers often use inexpensive and poorly absorbed nutrients. This low absorption rate is primarily due to 1) the poor absorption of the chemical source of the nutrient, and 2) nutrient-nutrient interactions.

With major pharmaceutical houses now joining the burgeoning supplement business, you can expect quality to decrease even further. In their business, the name of the game *is* business, and business *means* dollars. Manufacturers of products will compete with one another for shelf space in the large distribution company's locations. The manufacturer must do everything possible to meet the pricing needs of the major distribution chains.

Acquiring shelf space for a product in 5,000 K-Mart stores will boil down to one product selling for $5.99 versus another selling for $5.95. A product using the highest quality raw ingredients, but selling for $6.95, has no chance of placement because everyone involved in the marketing and distribution process understands that the consumer will buy on price and not quality. This is not because the consumer is unconcerned about quality, but because he does not possess the requisite knowledge to distinguish between products and the marketing claims made about them.

So the marketing machine simply states that the product they are selling is the best (even though it is not), and the consumer, believing this claim, can now make their choice based on a single criteria: the lowest price. That's an easy choice to make because if one is presented with two products of similar quality, they will always buy the least expensive one!

And the end result will be that you may save some money by

using these poorly manufactured nutritional supplements, but you will compromise your preventative efforts against disease.

When you add these two major changes to 1) poorly balanced formulas that use inappropriate combinations of nutrient supplements, 2) diets high in refined foods such as sugar and refined grains, and 3) nutrient-depleted foods from low-nutrient content soils, you have the potential for significant health problems. You must be very careful choosing the supplements that you will put into you body.

Colloidal Minerals

One of the hottest nutritional supplement rages of the late 1990's is colloidal minerals. In 1994, Dr. Joel Wallach, ND, released an audiotape called *Dead Doctors Don't Lie*. The tape promoted the benefits of colloidal minerals. Multi-level companies rose from the barren earth like skyscrapers touting the benefits of using these minerals. During the last four years, I have received more than 100 of these tapes through the mail soliciting me to purchase the product.

Colloidal minerals are claimed to prevent a variety of common illnesses arising from mineral deficiencies. But colloidal supplementation is a hotly debated topic. Are these minerals safe to take? Do they live up to the marketing claims?

Colloidal is a chemical term describing a substance containing particles so small that they remain in suspension in liquid or gas. Even though they're minuscule, colloidal particles, unlike dissolved particles and suspensions, retain their whole form. Colloidal minerals are derived from the clay of ancient seabeds. Their mineral composition varies depending on their origin. A single bottle of colloidal product could contain anywhere from one to nearly 100 minerals.

The great interest in supplementing with colloidal minerals is grounded in the theory that the wide variety of human health problems, the source of which lies in mineral deficiencies, would be more effectively treated with the more readily absorbable liquid colloidal form of minerals.

Proponents of colloidal minerals claim that this form of minerals are better absorbed than solid mineral forms because the molecules are small enough to pass through the intestinal lining. Therefore, the body does not to need break colloids down further in the digestive tract; they absorb as they are. Rates of absorption are critical in mineral nutrition. Even though a supplement contains a full quantity of the needed mineral, a low absorption rate decreases the amount of mineral delivered to the necessary site, the cell. This compromises any potential health benefits of mineral supplementation.

Wallach argues that colloidal forms are 98% absorbed compared with a much lower rate of absorption from other sources of essential minerals. No part of the colloidal discussion is as fraught with disagreement as that of absorption. Supporters, like Wallach, argue that colloidal minerals are better absorbed than other forms of minerals, but opponents, such as Tim Birdsall, ND, editor-in-chief of *Alternative Medical Review* disagrees. Dr. Birdsall states, "… the term colloidal actually infers nothing about the absorption or use of a substance by the body, it only describes whether a substance stays in solution or falls out of suspension."

Colloidal minerals are, by definition, small enough to remain in suspension, but are too large to pass through cell membranes, according to Taber's Medical Dictionary, 13th edition. "No one knows for sure if particle size is an issue because we need more research on the subject," says Bruce Woolley, PhD, professor of nutrition and pharmacology at Brigham Young University, Provo, Utah.

Supporters also claim that colloids are negatively charged, making them attractive to the positively charged intestinal lining. Opponents say this is preposterous. Alexander Schauss, PhD, director of the Life Science division of the American Institute for Biosocial Research in Tacoma, Washington, maintains that the small intestine's lining is actually negatively charged and would repel negatively charged colloidal clay particles.

In addition, Birdsall says that the 98% absorption rate claimed by Wallach is a scientifically unfounded and astounding figure, considering that minerals vary in absorption rates, with many absorbed from food at around the 10% rate.

Some colloidal minerals contain up to 90 minerals, far more than the established 15 essential minerals for good health. "There are only 109 elements in the periodic table, and if you subtract out the gases, heavy metals, and radioactive elements, there aren't 90 left that are good for you," says Woolley. "There's no research proving the safety of taking many of the minerals found in colloidal products."

Last year, Schauss analyzed 23 colloidal products and discovered that the levels of some minerals in colloidal products were so low that a person could obtain more trace elements for less money by drinking a glass of tap water. He tested the levels of 37 minerals, that all colloidal products claimed to contain, and found that, on average, the products contained only 13 of 37 minerals claimed.

Today, no human trials on the safety or efficacy of colloidal minerals exist.

Currently, the National Nutritional Foods Association, a natural products trade organization, is examining the safety and efficacy of colloidal products. It recommends that you insist on documentation from colloidal manufacturers: certificates of analysis from an independent laboratory stating the product's composition and listing the laboratory's address, phone number, and analyst's name. However, that does not change the fact that there are no studies about the potential health benefits provided by colloidal minerals.

Minerals are essential for good health. Dr. Henry Shroeder, Professor Emeritus at Dartmouth University (The Poisons Around Us, Keats Publishing) states "that minerals are far more important than vitamins." Based on many years of research, many scientists have shown that we need a minimum amount of minerals in our diet each day to provide our body with these essential nutrients. Today's diets are woefully low in essential minerals; supplementation is necessary.

The Reference Dietary Intake for key minerals is:

Mineral	Mg/Day (RDI)
Calcium	800-1,200*
Magnesium	280 F*; 350* M
Iron	15*
Manganese	2.0-5.0*
Zinc	12*
Chromium	0.2*
Selenium	0.05*
Copper	1.5-3.0*

* Depends on chemical source of minerals: amino acid chelate absorption is high and daily intake can be less to receive more.

Table 10.

In my view, there are two extremely important issues about colloidal minerals that one must consider before supplementing with these products:

1) **Quantity**: that is, how many milligrams of mineral are contained in a daily dose? You need a certain amount (quantity) of minerals in a daily dose. Colloidal mineral formulations contain minute quantities of minerals. Our bodies need milligrams of essential minerals each day. The content of minerals in colloidal minerals is so low that they can not be measured on a milligram scale! If one relied on these products for his sole source of daily mineral nutrition, he would surely begin to experience mineral deficiencies and the health problems attending nutrient deficiencies,

2) **Toxicity**: many of the metals in colloidal minerals are highly toxic in minute doses: ***beryllium*** and ***antimony*** are two highly poisonous metals that are listed as ingredients in colloidal minerals, and they should be avoided at all cost.

The main points in the paragraph above are that:

1) One must ingest a minimum quantity of minerals each day. This quantity ranges from a low of about 0.2 milligrams for chromium to 1,000 milligrams for calcium. Colloidal mineral formulations do not meet these requirements (they're not even close!)

2) Colloidal mineral solutions contain toxic heavy metals that you do not want in your body, in any amount. These toxic metals may slowly accumulate in the tissues of your body, even from the very small amounts contained in colloidal minerals.

It's your choice, but don't make that choice based upon the hogwash purveyed by Dr. Joel Wallach in his tape *Dead Doctor's Don't Lie*, or upon any other statements made by multi-level marketing hype of useless and possibly dangerous products. I always recommend to my clients that they stay far away from today's commercially available colloidal minerals.

chapter 7

Vitamins

The chemical sources for most vitamins are well absorbed. For vitamin C the most common source is ascorbic acid which is well absorbed. A new form of vitamin C is Ester-C. The manufacturer claims that it is better absorbed and more effectively used by the body's cells than ascorbic acid. Independent research, however, shows that Ester-C is no better absorbed than ascorbic acid. In fact, subjects tested for vitamin C content in their blood after the administration of both forms had higher blood levels when given ascorbic acid than when given Ester-C. This is just another example (of many) of marketing hoopla that doesn't stand the test of research.

In the family of B vitamins, some exciting new substances are in the marketplace. As ingredients in multivitamin and mineral supplements, they add significantly to the cost of the product, but the extra money you pay is worth it. Unfortunately it is very difficult, if not impossible, to find a major marketer of supplements who will use these powerful products.

Niacin (vitamin B_3) functions in the body as a part of two important coenzymes: NAD and NADP. These enzymes are involved in the body's energy cycle and its use of food as fuel. In the early 1900's many people died of a disease called pellagra. This disease is characterized by the 3-D's—dermatitis (the skin cracks and becomes scaly), dementia (the brain does not function properly leading to confusion), and diarrhea (the body fails to manufacture an adequate amount of mucus that protects the cells of the gastrointestinal tract).

The refining of grain products, with the consequent loss of niacin, led to a dietary deficiency of niacin in people's diets. This was the cause of the disease. This discovery of a niacin deficiency in flour, led to the mandatory food enrichment programs in which niacin was added back to refined flour. Today, niacin has reached a level of cult status, and niacin is used therapeutically to lower cholesterol and is given to patients suffering from arthritis. Scientific studies confirm the efficacy of niacin in the treatment of these conditions.

Vitamin B3 is available in nutritional supplements as either niacin (nicotinic acid or nicotinate) or niacinamide (nicotinamide). Many people supplement with high doses of niacin with intake levels exceeding 1,500 mg per day. These high doses of niacin cause a transient flushing of the skin (called the niacin flush), usually beginning on the forehead and moving down into the chest. This is only uncomfortable, but not dangerous.

Manufacturers have turned to timed-release capsules to avoid this problem, but there is a significant side effect: liver damage. A recent study in the *Journal of the American Medical Association* (JAMA) strongly recommended that timed-release niacin be restricted. In the study, 52% of the test subjects developed liver damage compared with none taking the immediate-release niacin.

A form of niacin, inositol hexanicotinate, has proven to be a vast improvement over currently available forms of niacin. This product has a strong track record of safe and successful use in Europe during the past 30 years. This form is well absorbed and provides a significantly more powerful biochemical and physiological effect than current niacin forms, but without the side effects of other forms of niacin.

Another B vitamin, pantothenic acid (B5), is very important in the use of food as energy. B5 is also useful to support the adrenal gland and joint function. It has long been considered the "anti-stress" vitamin because of its influence on adrenal function and cellular energy metabolism.

Pantothenic acid is available generally as calcium pantothenate, but the most active form is pantethine. Pantethine is very useful in cholesterol and triglyceride control. These are reputed to be two pre-eminent risk factors for heart disease. Pantethine is effective in lowering cholesterol and triglycerides, but pantothenic acid is not. There are no toxic effects or side effects from the use of pantethine.

As expected, for such a high-quality nutrient, pantethine is very expensive compared with other sources of B5. Major manufacturers will not source it for inclusion in their multi-vitamin and mineral supplement. In fact, you usually only find it as a stand-alone product because of the expense. But, it is so effective and such an advanced form of B5 supplementation that it makes a great deal of sense to include it as a regular ingredient in your supplement program—if you can find it.

Two other B vitamins that are commercially available in super forms are vitamin B2 (riboflavin) and vitamin B6 (pyridoxine).

Riboflavin-5-phosphate is the activated form of riboflavin and yields increased effectiveness versus the standard form provided in the majority of nutritional supplements.

Vitamin B6 is available as pyridoxine hydrochloride and pyridoxal-5-phosphate. Pyridoxal-5-phosphate is the most active form. Normally, the liver must convert pyridoxine to pyridoxal-5-phosphate, using riboflavin and magnesium as co-factors in the chemical conversion. As long as liver function is adequate, pyridoxine is OK to use. But if liver function is sub-optimal, then the use of the most active form as pyridoxal-5-phosphate may help in providing the body with more of the usable nutrient.

Today, with all the environmental pollution that exists and the amount of medicines used by adults and children alike, the liver is working overtime to detoxify or inactivate many of these man-made chemicals. It is very difficult to maintain optimal liver function. Using supplement ingredients that are the most active forms assures nutrient delivery to the cells. This added insurance is worth the price. Now, the only problem is to find a supplement formulator and manufacturer willing to go the extra mile to produce a quality product containing these specialized nutrients.

Vitamin K is another essential nutrient that too few manufacturers put into their multi-vitamin product. The primary health effects of vitamin K are in the maintenance of the blood's clotting ability. Vitamin K also helps to maintain the calcium content of the bones. Its principal use as a dietary supplement is in the prevention of osteoporosis and excessive menstrual bleeding. The most effective form is vitamin K1 (phylloquinone). Look for that as the source of vitamin K in your supplement—if, that is, your supplement even contains vitamin K.

chapter 8

Tissue Retention of Nutrients and Nutrient Interactions

Once a nutrient is absorbed from the gut, it must travel in the blood and enter the cell (muscle cell, brain cell, eye cell, etc.). This is called tissue uptake. The cell will use the nutrient to build new cell components and to carry-on the metabolic functions of the cell. The issue is now one of retention of the nutrient within the cell versus absorption from the gut.

Chelated minerals are an excellent source, compared with other chemical sources of minerals, for providing the raw mineral building blocks to maintain cell function.

The following graph shows how much calcium was retained in different tissues seven days after administration. The animal's tissues retained 54.4% more calcium when the source was an amino acid chelate versus the calcium source as calcium chloride.

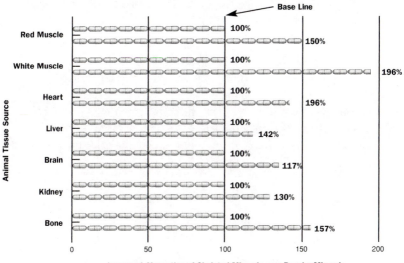

Graph 5. Amino acid chelates have a higher uptake into body tissues than minerals coming from other sources. In this graph, the uptake by body tissues, when provided with a poor chemical

source of mineral, served as a reference point setting of 100%. The graph shows the increased percent tissue uptake when the chemical source is pure amino acid chelate.

Balance of Nutrients: Particularly Minerals (the most important part of your supplement program)

Nutrient:Nutrient Interactions

The interactions between nutrients, particularly minerals, are another important aspect of nutrient supplementation. One might wonder why an understanding of the relationship between requirements for, and toxicity of, essential trace elements (minerals) is important. Essential trace elements are available over-the-counter. Because essential trace elements are nutrients, many people assume that if a little bit is good, more will be better, and therefore self-medicate themselves.

If Paracelsus' dictum, "the dose makes the poison," were more widely understood, self-medication might be less frequent. Toxic effects of essential trace elements have been known for many years from research in farm and experimental animals. Until recently, it had been assumed that the body's homeostatic (balance-maintaining) mechanisms effectively protected the body against excess amounts of most essential trace elements.

Particularly important is the concept of the spectrum of trace element nutrition: the spectrum ranges from 1) deficient, to 2) marginally adequate, to 3) fully adequate, to 4) marginally excessive, to 5) toxic. Students of nutrition will find little information clarifying the maximum safe dose of essential trace elements. This subject is poorly understood, yet it is of paramount importance to any person who regularly uses nutritional supplements.

Essential trace elements, that are similar in their chemistry, compete for attachments to other chemicals inside the body. Errors in the binding of the correct nutrient with another essential nutrient can impair body function.

Zinc to Copper Ratio as an Illustration of the Toxicity of Essential Trace Elements

This concept is exemplified by the zinc to copper ratio (Zn:Cu). The antagonism existing between these two essential trace elements was outlined long ago through the work of Dr. Leslie Klevay of the USDA Nutrition Research Center in South Dakota. Intestinal absorption of copper is inhibited by zinc. Therefore, the risk of copper deficiency is increased when a person ingests (or swallows a pill containing) a high level of zinc relative to the amount copper ingested.

Health problems caused by an imbalance between these two nutrients include decreased red blood cell copper and zinc superoxide dismutase. This chemical is very important in preventing free radical damage to the cell membranes and to the cell's metabolic machinery. An increased Zn:Cu ratio also decreases high density lipoprotein cholesterol. High-density lipoprotein cholesterol is the good cholesterol and individuals with high amounts of high-density lipoprotein are considered to have a reduced risk for heart disease. Other functional deficits from an imbalance in the Zn:Cu ratio include an inability to clear blood sugar, a reduction in immune system function, and abnormal heart function.

The work by Dr. Klevay over the last 25 years has consistently shown the negative health impact of too much zinc and too little copper. Deleterious health effects begin to show up when the Zn:Cu ratio exceeds 10 milligrams (mg) of zinc to 1 mg of copper. Dr. Klevay states that we have an absolute requirement for about 2 mg of copper per day. Unfortunately, the public's attention has been drawn to the importance of zinc for a myriad of health requirements including the common cold, skin problems, and the prostate gland in males.

As a result, people are self-supplementing with very high doses of zinc and seriously disturbing the delicate balance between zinc and copper. 50% of all Americans now take nutritional supplements. They use a wide array of products, many of which overload the use of zinc and, literally, pay no attention to the copper in the formulation. Users of these products face a significant health risk.

I have analyzed hundreds of nutritional supplements over the years, and it is rare indeed that a product has the proper balance and quantity of these two essential trace elements: zinc and copper. Most often, the amount of copper is woefully deficient and the amount of zinc is dangerously high.

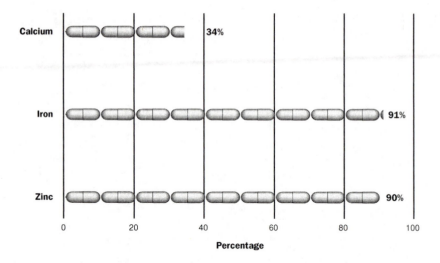

Calcium		34%			
Iron					91%
Zinc					90%

0   20   40   60   80   100

Percentage

Graph 6. Misuse of supplements: this chart shows the percent of people supplementing with zinc (and iron and calcium) without using the other balancing minerals. Zinc supplements without copper are dangerous.

This point is so important that Dr. Klevay has argued that it is the balance of the Zn:Cu ratio that is the primary risk factor for heart disease. By manipulating the Zn:Cu ratio in laboratory studies, he has induced all of the risk factors that doctors and scientists have attributed to the causes of heart disease. His research implies, and shows, that any abnormality in blood fats comes, not from diet (eating fat and cholesterol), but from a too-high Zn:Cu ratio and a too-low total copper intake.

It is not uncommon for supplement users to ingest more than 50 mg of zinc each day. Copper intake in many users of supplements is marginal or nonexistent. Daily copper intake from the typical diet of people living in the United States is about 0.8 mg/day. Zn:Cu ratios exceeding 20:1 are not uncommon. I have, in my analysis of many nutritional supplements, found supplement programs where the Zn:Cu ratio exceeds 70:1. One client even suffered a heart attack. His medical doctor never considered an imbalance between zinc to copper as a primary factor inducing his heart attack. I did.

Copper and Osteoporosis

Recent writings by Dr. Klevay noted that the 10th edition of Recommended Dietary Allowances (RDA) did not include a RDA for

52

copper; but rather a safe and adequate daily intake was suggested. He is disturbed by this omission because bone disease and cardiovascular disease resulting from diets low in copper have been known and studied in animals for decades.

Men and women fed diets containing about 1 mg of copper per day, amounts quite frequent in the US and considered marginal, responded similarly to copper deficient animals and experienced potentially harmful changes in blood pressure control, cholesterol and glucose metabolism, and electrocardiograms.

Women using a supplement containing trace elements that included copper experienced beneficial effects on bone density. The association between osteoporosis and low copper intake is strong. A high intake of zinc relative to copper is also a significant risk factor for osteoporosis.

These results in using copper as a key nutritional supplement are more impressive than results experienced by subjects supplementing with magnesium, selenium, and zinc. Heart disease and osteoporosis are likely consequences of diets low in copper, the typical diet consumed by the US population.

Dr. Klevay states that, "Committees that establish RDA's should return to earlier traditions of editions of the Recommended Dietary Allowances and make recommendations that promote health and nutritional welfare, meet functional needs, and prevent disease and promote public welfare." Strong statements indeed.

A recent study determined the ideal amount of supplemental zinc that would provide an adequate intake at a safe dose. This comprehensive study considered the absorption of zinc and copper from the intestinal tract so that an accurate assessment of the total intake was included in the analysis.

For the average bodyweight individual, the over-the-counter dose that was considered safe was 9 mg per day. This amount was established as the reference dose for a 60-kilogram (132 pound) adult. Based on this evaluation, almost all over-the-counter zinc supplements are **unsafe** (emphasis added).

Note that the researcher chose his words very carefully. He says that almost all over-the-counter zinc supplements are unsafe; not a casual too much, but unsafe. That also means toxic and dangerous.

The researcher concluded his article by stating that self-medication with zinc might not be a good idea.

Other nutrient:nutrient interactions that reduce nutrient bioavailability include vitamin D with calcium and interactions between copper, molybdenum, and sulphur. Vitamin C also affects the nutritional availability of iron. Ascorbic acid (vitamin C) slows and impairs the absorption of copper from the intestinal tract in several animal models studied.

These are several examples of how nutrients interact with one another. I do not believe that it is prudent to take a casual attitude towards nutritional supplementation programs. There are a tremendous number of poorly designed nutritional supplements on the market. From the research of many scientists, we know that individuals can suffer from serious disease processes because of mineral imbalances. Interactions of both vitamins and minerals with one another should be a serious concern when choosing a daily supplement of essential nutrients.

And the more you supplement in a random fashion, buying a bottle of this and a bottle of that, the more dangerous your program becomes.

More is not always better. And a shotgun approach to product design, as most companies follow, is far from ideal. Danger lurks; just ask my client who had the heart attack.

That's why it is so important to pay attention to the supplements that you use: your first consideration should be that the supplement contains all of the essential nutrients and that they are in the right balance with one another. The second, yet just as important, consideration is the quality of the chemical sources of the nutrients in your tablets or capsules. They should be of the highest quality to assure you that you will reap the best possible reward from the supplement's use.

Nutrient:Toxin Interactions

Dr. Henry Schroeder, Professor emeritus at Dartmouth College, has stated, "that the five toxic trace metals—cadmium, mercury, lead, beryllium, and antimony—are extremely important to the health of the public being involved in at least half the deaths in the US and much of the disabling disease."

The EPA has set an upper safe limit for lead at 10 mg/dL (milligrams per deciliter—a volume of blood). The previous upper safe limit for lead was 25 mg/dL. Research over the years has shown that the level of 25 mg/dL was too high. The EPA has further lowered the safe limit to 10 mg/dL. During the years that the upper limit was set at 25 mg/dL, the average lead content in the blood of American citizens was 12 mg/dL. Therefore, for many years, if we use the current standard, the majority of Americans suffered from a too high blood concentration of lead. And lead is a nasty actor causing all kinds of health problems that are blamed on other causes.

Recent research, in the late 1980's and the early 1990's, has shown that lead concentrations in the blood as little as 1 mg/dL have led to neurological (brain) damage in laboratory animals. The average concentration of lead in the blood of American citizens today is approximately 3 mg/dL. It doesn't take an Einstein to figure the potential hazards from our current day levels.

Lead, cadmium, and mercury are toxic metals that are non-essential for our nutritional needs. The toxic effects of these metals may be mediated or enhanced by interactions or deficiencies of nutritionally essential metals. Lead competes with calcium and replaces it in critical cellular functions. Important functional changes include the inhibition of the release of neurotransmitters in the brain and nervous system and interference with the regulation of cell metabolism by binding to calcium receptors.

Dietary deficiencies of calcium, iron, and zinc increase the effects of lead on cognitive and behavioral development. Iron deficiency increases the gastrointestinal absorption of cadmium, and cadmium competes with zinc for binding sites on metallothionein, which is important in the storage and transport of zinc during development.

An exciting area of thinking today is that of sub-clinical toxicity. This is the idea that one doesn't necessarily have to contract cancer to suffer from the toxic effects of chemical elements. The thought underlying the concept of sub-clinical toxicity is that the damaging agent can begin to decrease bodily function at much lower levels of concentration than those which lead to cancer.

As you can see, this is a complex issue, and there are a high number of interactions between different nutrients and between nutrients and toxic substances. I covered in detail the interaction between the Zn:Cu ratio. The interaction between calcium and lead is a significant nutrient:toxin interaction as well. Dr. David A. McCarron, co-founder of the Calcium Information Center, has stated that half of all

Americans, males and females, are "consuming an inadequate amount of calcium."

I have already outlined the significant deficiencies existing in many Americans' dietary nutrient intakes since the first surveys were conducted in the late 1960's. The surveys have consistently demonstrated an inadequate intake of nutrients across both sexes and in all age groups. This fact alone should alarm all citizens for themselves and for their families. However, today, there is a confounding factor that increases the danger of a poor diet: that is the level of environmental pollution. Environmental pollution is a significant stressing agent to the body's effort to maintain health.

Therefore, it is essential that one ingest, not only an adequate intake of all the essential nutrients to meet previously defined needs, but also to achieve an optimal intake as insurance against the ever-increasing effects of pollution and stress.

chapter 9

Understanding Antioxidants

One of the hottest revenue makers in the multi-billion dollar nutritional supplement industry in the 1990's revolves around antioxidant nutritional supplements. Antioxidants protect against free radical damage. Scientific research is now relating specific diseases to oxidation and damage to body systems by free radicals. Examples of these diseases include Alzheimer's, atherosclerosis, diabetes, cancer, emphysema, malaria, muscular dystrophy, Parkinson's disease, rheumatoid arthritis, and retinal degeneration.

As I have stated previously, the theme of this monograph and its intended goal are to help you choose a <u>basic</u> nutritional supplement containing all of the <u>essential</u> nutrients. With that in mind, I will discuss the role and purpose of antioxidant supplementation and how you can best benefit by proper and appropriate supplementation with antioxidants.

I want to present a comprehensive picture of antioxidant nutritional supplementation and sources of antioxidants from the diet. However, to do this properly requires a certain amount of detail that some readers might find too technical and too cumbersome. So first, I will present a basic primer that is the **Short Version,** and, following that, I will present the **Long** (more technical) **Version** (for those who are interested in more technical information).

Antioxidants: Short Version

Free radicals are formed by the body cells as they breakdown food to release stored energy from the food to do the mechanical and chemical work of the body. Free radicals, in excessive quantities, can damage the body's genetic material, immune system, and the cell membranes that maintain the integrity of our organs and systems and, ultimately, our total health.

Antioxidants counteract the damaging action of free radicals and prevent any potential damage that the free radicals might create. The primary source of antioxidants is the food we eat. The principal antioxidants in food sources are located within the fat of both plants and animals. An additional source of necessary antioxidant compounds is animal protein.

There are two types of antioxidants: those that are fat-soluble and those that are water-soluble. The body's **First Line of Defense** against free radicals in the **Antioxidant Defense System** is contained within the fat layer of all cell and cellular membranes. The **Second Line of Defense** is in the aqueous or water-phase area of the cell. This point, that of two lines of defense in the body's antioxidant strategy, is critical for your understanding of antioxidant nutrients and will allow you to make appropriate dietary and nutritional supplement choices.

The primary nutrients in the **First Line of Defense** include vitamin Q (CoQ10), vitamin E, and vitamin C. The **Second Line of Defense** includes various bioflavonoids such as vitamin P and other phytochemicals (plant based, herb-like chemicals).

It is now well accepted among scientific researchers that an adequate intake of antioxidants is essential to good health. Many authorities recommend that, in addition to one's daily diet, one ingest an appropriate nutritional supplement. It is very difficult, in today's nutritional marketplace, abounding with hyped-up claims, to know exactly what supplements to choose.

An appropriate antioxidant supplement should include vitamin Q, vitamin E, and vitamin C, along with selenium. Vitamin A, particularly as beta-carotene, should also be a part of the basic supplement program. These nutritional items are the critical components in the body's antioxidant strategy. Additional components, such as the bioflavonoid Pycnogenol, make up the **Second Line of Defense** in the body's antioxidant strategy and are not considered as a part of the primary supplement.

Therefore, if a manufacturer decreases the amount of essential nutrients in a capsule or tablet to make room for a small amount of Pycnogenol, the supplement now short-changes the consumer with too little amounts of both the primary antioxidants <u>and</u> the secondary antioxidants.

Current emphasis on nutritional supplements such as Pycnogenol over-emphasize its role in the body's antioxidant strategy at the expense of the most essential nutrients, including vitamin C, vitamin Q, and vitamin E. Vitamin Q is very expensive and therapeutic doses of 30 milligrams or more add a significant cost if it were a part of a comprehensive, basic nutritional supplement.

It is impossible to find a basic nutritional supplement containing all the essential nutrients described earlier in this monograph that also contains many of the newer, specialized nutrients coming into the marketplace today. Much of today's marketing strategy focuses on antioxidants, but much of that marketing is misplaced, and you, as the consumer, end up buying a jar of pine bark extract which contains antioxidants only from the **Second Line of Defense**.

There you are. That's the short primer on antioxidants. For more detailed information, read the next section. If the notion of immersing yourself in a more detailed discussion threatens to bore you, then you'll find information about the appropriate selection of quantities of the various antioxidant nutrients at the end of the **Long Version** section.

Antioxidants: Long Version

The primary function of antioxidants is to grab-up dangerous free radicals that are produced as a result of cellular metabolism. We must answer two important questions:

1) What are free radicals and how are they produced?

2) What are antioxidants and how do they protect us against free radical damage?

Production of Free Radicals: As the body breaks down ingested food into smaller and smaller molecules, the food particles travel through a long chain of chemical steps made possible by a wide array of enzymes whose job is to transform the food into a form usable by the body. During this process, stored energy is unleashed from the food, and it is this energy that the body's cells use to do the work of that organ (kidney, liver, and muscles, etc.) or system (immune system).

The fancy biochemical name for the chemical process of breaking food down to release energy is called **reduction-oxidation reactions**. During the process of reduction-oxidation reactions, electrons (these are the key carriers of energy inside the cell) are shuttled from one place to the next inside the cell.

As this movement occurs, energy flows out at each successive step providing the currency necessary to power the cell's metabolic activities. During this process, the formation of the dangerous free radicals occurs.

Under normal cellular conditions, free radicals are disposed of as quickly as they are formed. But under stressful conditions, such as vigorous exercise or disease, free radicals may accumulate faster than they can be disposed.

A free radical is a chemical with one, or several, unpaired electrons in its outer electron orbit. (If you do not understand this, you aren't alone. Don't worry about it; I included this for people who have a technical interest in these kinds of things.) The unpaired electron is extremely reactive, which is the chemical and physical reason for the reactivity of the free radical.

The point to remember is this: it is these unpaired electrons floating around in the cell that are hazardous.

The next important (most important) point to understand is the location, in the cell, where all this activity occurs. To help you visualize what I am about to describe, first, picture in your mind, a tennis ball. Imagine that the covering of the tennis ball is the same as the outer covering of any one of the cells in your body. This covering provides protection from environmental threats. It also allows nutrients and waste products to selectively pass in and out of the cell: it is selectively porous. It is the gate-keeper and protective barrier to the all-important interior of the cell.

Now, picture the inside of the cell: here, instead of air as is in the tennis ball, there is a factory with thousands of workers, all performing the work of the cell, such as filtering for liver cells, seeing for eye cells, and thinking for brain cells. The factory workers inside the cell also have a covering similar to the covering of the tennis ball. Therefore, each cell is made up of its outer, protective covering, and workers inside the cell also have their own outer, protective covering. Each part, however, is dependent on the other for its protection and nourishment. The coverings of these different compartments protect their interiors from outside dangers.

The coverings of both the cell and the smaller parts inside the cell are made up of proteins and fats. Another word used by scientists for fats is lipids. The proteins and lipids are layered around the cell membrane and around the cell parts—one on top of the other. This is called the lipid-protein bi-layer. There is a center lipid layer with a protein layer on either side of it like a cheese sandwich: two pieces of bread with a slice of cheese in between.

The cells that make up an organ or system have common functions. The cells that make up different organs or systems have functions specific to the work of that organ or system. Regardless of the extreme difference in cellular functions, according to the organ or system in which they are located, there is one feature that is common to all cells: they must have energy to do the work of the cell. And this energy comes from the food we eat. Food must combine with the oxygen we breathe in order for the body to extract the energy from the food. Together, the food and oxygen produce the energy required by the cell to perform its tasks. The final step in the production of energy from food occurs inside the cell and is absolutely dependent on a supply of oxygen.

The oxygen that we breathe is essential to life on earth. The organelle inside the cell where energy production occurs is called the mitochondria. In the process of producing energy, oxygen combines with some of the unpaired electrons and forms free radicals. Free radicals are constantly formed within the outer cell membrane, within the mitochondria (in the interior of the cell), and within other interior cellular components.

Under normal conditions, free radical formation in the cell is very aggressively and actively kept under control by the **Antioxidant Defense System**. This is also known as the **Antioxidant Strategy** of the cell. It is important to understand that the majority of free radicals are formed in the lipid layer of cell membranes. This includes the lipids that form the outer cell wall and the lipids forming the membranes of mitochondria and other cellular organelles. So, the free radical formation, and the process of their disposal, occurs *inside* the piece of cheese that is "sandwiched" between the two pieces of bread.

This grabbing-up process of free radicals that the **Antioxidant Defense System** performs is known as *scavenging* or *quenching*. Most free radicals exist only during a fraction of a second before they have participated in another chemical reaction freeing the cell from the ever-present danger created by free radical formation.

The lipid (fat) layer of the cellular membranes contains the enzymes that are necessary for the chemical reactions that produce free radicals. So, it is here that the battle against free radical damage is won or lost. The primary nutrients that scavenge and quench the free radicals are also located in the lipid layer. These nutrients are lipophilic (fat-loving) and are designed to hang-out in the fat layer where they can destroy the free radicals.

In contrast to the fat-loving nutrients, other antioxidants reside only *partly* in the lipid layer of the membranes or *fully* in the water layer in the interior of the cell. The nutrients that mix only in the water layer of the cell are called hydrophilic (water-loving).

All antioxidants are natural compounds that are found in foods. The principal antioxidant vitamins and minerals are vitamin A, vitamin Q (also called ubiquinone and CoQ10), vitamin C, vitamin E, vitamin P (bioflavonoids), zinc, and selenium.

The major **lipophilic** or fat-loving nutrients are vitamin Q, vitamin E, and beta-carotene. Together, these lipophilic antioxidant vitamins make up the **First Defense Line**. A **Secondary Defense Line** includes the water-soluble vitamin C, several members of the vitamin B group, vitamin P, and an additional antioxidant enzyme system represented by glutathione and glutathione peroxidase and reductase.

It is of critical importance in selecting your daily nutritional supplement to understand the above distinctions: *some nutrients within the cell are fat-loving and some nutrients are water-loving*. Both types are important in the body's antioxidant strategy. But it is the fat-loving nutrients that are of primary importance and represent the **First Line of Defense** for the cell's antioxidant system.

Remember this pecking order and make sure that your supplement contains adequate amounts of the **First Defense Line** of antioxidant nutrients. Concentrating on a nutritional supplement that contains nutrients that are active only in the **Second Line of Defense** is a mistake; they (the **Second Line of Defense** antioxidants) can act maximally only if the lipid layer is well saturated with the fat-loving antioxidant nutrients.

Radical Formation and Cell Protection: The Antioxidant Strategy

Reactive free radicals must be controlled and stopped from reaching cellular components such as lipids, proteins, and other complicated molecules, such as the genetic material (DNA and RNA). These molecules and cellular chemicals immediately react with a free radical, and they can become more or less permanently rearranged, fragmented, or destroyed. Sometimes, cellular membranes and cell parts can be permanently and irreversibly destroyed.

The antioxidant strategy of the cell is based on the fact that, with few exceptions, the major free radical formation occurs in the lipid layers of cell membranes, including the inner cellular organelle's lipid membranes. The free radical is then transferred to the water-soluble compartments inside the cell. The lipid (fat)-soluble antioxidants (the lipophilic antioxidants) are vitamin Q, vitamin E, and vitamin C. These are the critical parts of the free radical fighting system and are referred to collectively as the Q-E-C cycle.

Vitamin Q, vitamin E, vitamin A, and beta-carotene are soluble primarily in lipids and lipid structures. As stated previously, the nutrients of the **First Line of Defense** are located in the lipid membrane coverings. Many recent studies have found that the fat-loving antioxidant vitamins Q and E are interrelated. Vitamin Q affects vitamin E and stimulates the chemical reactions in which vitamin E is involved.

However, one portion of the vitamin E molecule sticks out into the water layer of the cell. This distribution of vitamin E affects the antioxidant function in respect to vitamin Q and vitamin C. In the vitamin Q-E-C cycle, the electrons grabbed-up by vitamin Q in the scavenging process are transferred to vitamin E. These electrons are then transferred from vitamin E to vitamin C and other hydrophilic (water-loving) antioxidants such as vitamin P and glutathione.

In this way, vitamin C replenishes vitamin E so that it can continue scavenging free radicals within the lipid layer of the cell membrane. This is the interrelated action of the vitamin Q-E-C cycle.

Since Vitamin E is partially located within the lipid layer of the outer surface of cell membrane and *also* within the water area of the cell, it is more removed from the immediate, direct battle against free radical scavenging and quenching than is vitamin Q.

In this scenario, some of the cell's vitamin C pool is compartmentalized in both the lipid membranes, which surround the aqueous or water part of cell, and in the pure water area of the cell. Vitamin C enhances the action of the lipophilic or fat-loving antioxidant systems, primarily vitamin E and beta-carotene. The important interaction between vitamin Q, vitamin C, and vitamin E is essential to the cell's antioxidant strategy.

In most body tissues, the vitamin E concentration exceeds that of vitamin Q by 5 to 20 times. But, vitamin Q is a more potent quencher of free radicals than vitamin E because it can interact during the initial stages of free radical formation. This is because it is solely located within the lipid layer of the membrane where the bulk of free radical activity occurs. It is estimated that vitamin Q is 10 times stronger than vitamin E as an antioxidant, even though the concentration of vitamin E is significantly higher than that of vitamin Q.

The vitamin Q-E-C cycle is of primary importance in considering antioxidant supplementation and forms the basis for choosing a supplement that will provide the most bang-for-your-buck.

Chemical Structure and Types of Antioxidants

One of the basic chemical structures for molecules with strong free radical fighting properties is a carbon-ring structure. This carbon-ring structure has six sides (like an hexagon) and is known chemically as a phenol. These compounds are abundant in all living organisms. In biology and medicine, many phenol-based compounds are referred to as flavonoids (bioflavonoids, phytochemicals, or vitamin P). Theoretically, they are all capable of attracting free radicals.

Vitamin Q is also made up of a phenol ring. More often referred to in nutrition circles as CoQ10, vitamin Q is present in many foods and is available and absorbed as a nutrient. Under certain conditions, when the body is unable to manufacture adequate amounts of vitamin Q, it can potentially become a *conditionally essential nutrient*. However, international nutrition authorities have not yet recognized vitamin Q as an essential nutrient.

Scavenging and quenching power varies from one phenol species to another. Bioflavonoids, also called Vitamin P, are interesting molecules within the **Antioxidant Defense System**. Many researchers believe that vitamin P is an explanation for such phenomena as the health effects of the Mediterranean diet and the French paradox, in which red wine consumption, with its high concentration of phenols from grapes, seems to protect the French population from heart disease and other chronic diseases.

Plants and microorganisms are both able to manufacture phenol compounds. Animals do not have the necessary enzymes to manufacture them. One dietary source for phenol compounds is the essential amino acid phenylalanine. Phenylalanine is formed by plants and microorganisms and accumulates in animal protein. As a result, animal protein is the best source of these essential compounds for humans.

Many vitamins—such as vitamins Q, E, A, beta-carotene, and

K—are phenol structures. All of them participate in reduction-oxidation reactions. Today, antioxidant research has only scratched the surface in terms of the nutrients contained in food that act as antioxidants. It is most likely that the number of antioxidants yet to be discovered will equal in number the ones that are known today. One example is lipoic acid. This is another nutrient that is contained in foods, but supplementation has been shown to increase its action in providing health benefits.

In summary, many cellular chemicals have antioxidant properties. One of the primary chemical structures for antioxidants is the carbon-ring of a phenol compound. Current theories suggest that vitamin Q (CoQ10) is of primary importance. Vitamin Q is present in food, and the body is also able to manufacture it. However, sometimes food sources and the body manufacturing process provide too little of it to meet our needs.

Vitamin Q's central role is to feed electrons into the antioxidant defense machinery. Because the majority of free radicals are formed in the lipid layers of cell membranes, the first antioxidant defense line is that of the lipophilic or fat-loving antioxidants, vitamin Q and vitamin E. Vitamin E is present in much higher quantities than vitamin Q, but vitamin Q has higher antioxidant activity than vitamin E.

In the vitamin Q-E-C cycle, vitamin C frees vitamin E of its free radical load, thereby reconstituting fresh vitamin E in the lipid layer of the cell membranes. Vitamin Q increases the efficiency of vitamin E's antioxidant activity. Vitamin P, various phytochemicals, and the bioflavonoids provide important antioxidant activity. But it is important to remember that these bioflavonoid and phytochemical nutrients are not the **First Line of Defense**; they are, at best, a part of the **Second Line of Defense** in the body's fight against free radicals.

Antioxidant Activity of Flavonoids

Keeping in mind that the vitamin Q-E-C cycle is the **First Line of Defense** in the antioxidant strategy, we can now discuss some of the elements within the **Second Line of Defense**. Principal components include vitamin P whose chemical source is various phytochemicals (plants and herbs) and bioflavonoids. The protective effect of diets rich in fruits and vegetables has been attributed partly to the antioxidants contained in these foods.

Recent scientific work is beginning to highlight the potential role of these phenolic compounds. As stated above, phenolic compounds have a high potential for antioxidant activity and act as agents that may contribute to protection against heart disease and cancer. The bioflavonoids represent a large class of phytochemicals with free radical scavenging properties.

In selecting a nutritional supplement that provides antioxidant activity, it's important that you not succumb to the marketing hype. Claims by nutritional supplement manufacturers are, more often than not (far more often), untrue, wild exaggerations of the "nutritional superiority" of their products. With the increasing popularity of antioxidants, companies are rising from the desert sand shouting claims about the newest antioxidants.

Teas, wines, and fruit juices represent the most significant sources for the manufacture of antioxidant products sold today. Keep in mind, however, that these phytochemicals are involved <u>only</u> at the **Second Line of Defense** in the body's antioxidant strategy. They are not your most important sources for antioxidant supplementation and you should use them only after you are adequately nourished with the nutrients from the **First Line of Defense**.

The **Total Antioxidant Activity** of a nutrient (**TAA**) is measured by an antioxidant's ability to scavenge free radicals generated in both the lipophilic (fat) phase and in the aqueous (water) phase of a cell. The following table presents some values for common antioxidants that are marketed today either as foods or as nutritional supplements. The unit of measure is a **TEAC** (**Trolox Equivalent Antioxidant Activity**): this compares the antioxidant activity of the test bioflavonoid to the antioxidant activity of a known concentration of water-soluble vitamin E. Again, keep in mind that I'm discussing antioxidants that are part of the **Second Line of Defense** in the antioxidant strategy.

Relative Antioxidant Activity of Bioflavonoids

Antioxidant	Sources	TEAC
Flavonoids		
Anthocyanidins		
Oenin	Black grapes/red wine	1.8
Cyanidin	Grapes, raspberry, strawberry	4.4
Flavonols		
Quercetin	Onion, Apple skin, berries, black grapes, tea., broccoli	4.4
Kaempferol	Endive, leek, broccoli, grapefruit, tea	1.3
Flavone		
Rutin		2.4
Luteolin	Lemon, olive, celery, red pepper	2.1
Chrysin	Fruit skin	1.4
Apigenin	Celery, parsley	1.5
Flavonols		
Epicatechin	Black grapes/red wine	2.4
Epigallocatechin	Teas	3.8
Epigallocatechin gallate	Teas	4.8
Epicatechin gallate	Teas	4.9
Carotenoids		
Carotenes		
Lycopene	Tomatoes	2.9
Beta-carotene	Carrots, sweet potato, tomatoes, paprika, green veg.	1.9
Alpha-carotene	Tomatoes, carrots, green vegetables	1.3
Xanthophylls		
Beta-cryptoxanthin	Mango, papaya, peaches, paprika, oranges	2.0
Lutein	Banana, egg yolk, green vegetables	1.5
Zeaxanthin	Paprika	1.4
Canthaxanthin	Carrots, kale, red peppers	0.02

Table 11.

It is not important to memorize the chart; it is only important, however, that you understand, after reviewing the numbers, that there are methods to evaluate the claims made by marketers of nutritional supplements. Clearly, the concentration of some nutrients as a dried herb or as a concentrated herbal tincture will provide higher levels of antioxidant activity than many food sources. But, the point is this; there is a wide range of foods and nutritional supplements that are able to provide you with the nutrients you need. Armed with this information, you will not be fooled by the claims of the magical properties touted by the manufacturers.

Determining Your Optimal Intake of Antioxidant Nutrients

Determining the optimal intake and the correct balance of antioxidant nutrients is one of the greatest challenges in the nutrition and free radical field today. The significance of a mixed, well-balanced diet as the basis for successful nutritional therapy for daily living and in sports performance is obvious.

The **First Line of Defense** antioxidants, vitamin E and vitamin Q, are located within the fat compartment of plants and animals. Today's mania toward a low-fat diet has significantly compromised our intake of these primary antioxidant nutrients. This is particularly true for individuals who exercise regularly and for competitive athletes.

The high-carbohydrate diet that is in vogue today does not represent a balanced diet. Dr. Jan Karlsson, one of the original developers of the carbohydrate-loading regimen so popular among current-day athletes, has argued vehemently against a high-carbohydrate diet as a regular, everyday regimen. He claims that such a diet is only acceptable for two or, at most, four days within the framework of the carbohydrate and muscle glycogen loading program.

The carbohydrate-enriched diet leading to muscle glycogen loading has been widely accepted since the late 1960's as an important way to prepare for endurance sports and training. The dietary program, however, was to be applied *only occasionally*. Unfortunately, it was developed into a long-term treatment program and was used, not only by elite cross-country skiers and long-distance runners, but also by professional athletes in many different sports.

Even international organizations such as the International Olympic Committee Medical Commission recommended the use of the high-carbohydrate diet for athletes. *Dr. Karlsson has stated that such long-term dietary regimens are synonymous with malnutrition.* It has been shown that the intake of lipophilic nutrients such as vitamin E is linearly related to fat intake.

Other risks are associated with such an extreme high-carbo-hydrate diet if followed for a long time. In fact, this dietary regimen means that individuals may actually sacrifice their own structural lipids for energy needs. Vitamin Q and vitamin E are significant factors for the health of white blood cells; they're the cells that are richest in anti-oxidants and, consequently, enhance the immune system. Significant immune system suppression is a possible result of low dietary intake of fats and the consequent utilization of one's own fat stores as an energy source.

Athletes, with an extremely high intake of carbohydrates and, hence, subsequent impaired intake of lipid-based or lipophilic nutrients, have been in a situation referred to as the **Carbohydrate Syndrome** or the **Carbohydrate Trap**.

It seems reasonable to assume that this condition might reduce free radical elimination and lead to damage in muscles, increases in cell injury, and an inhibition of the body's inflammation and healing process in response to injury and infection. Hard-training athletes, who follow a high-carbohydrate diet, will suffer from overuse injuries due to a decreased ability to repair and rebuild damaged tissues. Vegetarians and others who consume a low-fat diet are also at serious risk for the same type of damage.

People who have extreme energy needs, such as athletes and those involved in manual labor, must be very careful about the sources of their daily food intake. If foods rich in carbohydrates come to serve as their primary source of energy, their risk of suffering from an insuffi-cient supply of nutrients will increase. Fats contain many of the essen-tial nutrients we need each day to maintain our health. As I have pro-posed for many years, the low-fat diet is dangerous.

Sports medicine authorities have just recently recognized the existence of the **Carbohydrate Trap** or *fat-phobia*. The **Carbohydrate Trap** represents a stage of malnutrition imposed by unprofessional advisors and followed by unwitting, unknowledgeable clients. This is one of the major difficulties in nutrition today: the emphasis on the low-fat diet in contrast to a diet that maintains an adequate fat intake. How long will it take until our medical and scientific "experts" recognize the folly of their recommendation of low-fat eating?

The prime objective, when embarking upon a nutritional supplement program, is to achieve satisfactory nourishment through a well-balanced diet.

Adding to a well-balanced diet, healthy people can achieve adequate blood concentrations of vitamin Q and vitamin E with a daily supplement of 50 to 100 mg of vitamin Q and 100 to 300 mg of vitamin E. This should be combined with a supplemental intake of 1,000 to 2,000 milligrams of vitamin C.

This supplement program is for the average person with a normal physical activity level. A higher level of physical activity demands an additional intake of these essential nutrients. For example, for elite endurance athletes, the program can be doubled (a 200% increase). In contrast to other lipophilic vitamins, such as vitamin A and vitamin D, high intakes of vitamin Q and vitamin E do not have significant side effects. Treatments of 300 to 400 mg of vitamin Q or of 1 to 2 grams of vitamin E have been given without any side effects.

One of the major problems in the nutritional supplement industry today is the notion that, if a little bit is good, then a lot is much better. In some instances, such as high doses of the vitamin B complex, side effects from over-dosing are minimal. However, this is not the case with minerals and several of the antioxidant compounds.

Because of all the hoopla surrounding the anti-aging and anti-disease benefits of antioxidant supplementation, people can easily overdose with these nutrients. Research studies estimate that each cell in the body suffers 10,000 free radical "hits" each day. The body's antioxidant supply is the basis of the antioxidant strategy against this potential damage. But, this defense isn't perfect. That's why free radical damage accumulates if conditions are not ideal to prevent it.

A relationship exists between free radicals and antioxidants; and they should be in balance to one another. One of the earliest workers who performed basic research in free radical theory was Dr. Denham Harman, MD, PhD. Dr. Harman's own supplement program at age 79 was: 200-400 IU of vitamin E, 2,000 mg of vitamin C, 100 micrograms of selenium, and 30 mg of vitamin Q (CoQ10) each day, plus 25,000 IU of beta-carotene every other day.

Dr. Harman was quoted in The Nutrition Reporter, "I'd take more, but I can't afford to be fatigued." He went on to explain that excessive antioxidants could cause fatigue and muscle weakness. He related the story of a person who regularly ingested 1,600 IU of vitamin E per day along with 100,000 IU of beta-carotene and an additional 50,000 IU of alpha-carotene. The subject suffered constantly from fatigue, but when he reduced his daily intake to less than half the level above, his fatigue evaporated.

Harman stated an important point: some experiments have shown that vitamin E supplements increase stamina; other experiments show that too high a dose decreases energy levels. There is a point of diminishing return. Again, one can never take a casual attitude toward his use of nutritional supplements.

In conclusion, how much antioxidant supplementation is required? There's no simple answer. The traditional, and low, Recommended Dietary Allowances (RDAs) are in a state of flux and will probably be revised upward. In 1995, the nonprofit Alliance for Aging Research recommended that generally healthy people take 100-400 IU of vitamin E, 200-1,000 mg of vitamin C, and 17,500-50,000 IU of beta-carotene daily to prevent many degenerative diseases. These values are quite consistent with those recommended by Dr. Jan Karlsson for generally healthy people, and will, with a slight adjustment upward, add a level of insurance to protect athletes in heavy training.

The key is to take enough antioxidants to slow the aging process and stave off degenerative diseases, but not so much that you become fatigued or compromise your immune system and other bodily functions.

Antioxidant nutritional supplementation is a bulwark in today's nutritional supplement products. Most important for the consumer is to select a product that contains the primary ingredients of the **First Line of Defense** in the body's antioxidant strategy. This includes vitamin Q (CoQ10), vitamin E, and vitamin C. In addition, the supplement should provide vitamin A, particularly as beta-carotene, and vitamin C. Ascorbic acid is an effective source for vitamin C supplementation. Next, an adequate amount of selenium (200 micrograms/day) should be an essential part of the supplement.

You may consider adding to your basic program a supplement of the **Second Line of Defense** antioxidant nutrients, including vitamin P, which come from bioflavonoids and various phytochemicals,. One of the hottest bioflavonoids today is called Pycnogenol, which is a pine bark extract. Pycnogenol is from a family of bioflavonoids called antho-

71

cyanidins. However, it is important not to become caught-up in the hype surrounding many of these products. Sure, many of them are very good, but don't get pulled into the marketing hype that a bottle of Pycnogenol tablets is going to cure you of the aging process and other chronic diseases.

Some supplement manufacturers are beginning to combine several different phytochemicals into one capsule or tablet. This is a good idea, as each phytochemical can provide additional free radical scavenging or quenching activity. However, if you review the table presented earlier in this section, you'll see that there are methods to validate scientifically the scavenging and quenching activity of individual phytochemicals. This information will serve as a basis for you to evaluate the sales and marketing messages bombarding you about individual nutritional supplements.

chapter 10

Nutritional Supplement Marketing Strategies

There is an explosion in nutritional supplement consumption, with almost 50% of all Americans ingesting supplements each day. Consumers purchase products through pharmacies, giant discount chain stores, multi-level companies, and supermarkets; marketing methods include television infomercials, radio advertising, and advice from "experts" of all types, including chiropractors, movie stars, doctors, pharmacists, and even the neighbor up the street. These represent some of the many channels of distribution for manufacturers of supplements.

In an attempt to capture a piece of the nutritional supplement market, manufacturers and distributors rely on consumers' lack of knowledge about nutritional supplements (of course, most manufacturers also suffer from a lack of knowledge about nutritional supplements). Three of the primary marketing strategies employed to induce customers to purchase products from a specific company and to win customer loyalty to that company and its products are:

1) **False Claims (masqueraded as the Truth)**: marketers design products and claim anything so that you will buy the products they produce—anything. I wish that this were not true, but it *is* true.

2) **Fear Tactic**: marketers design products for specific diseases or make claims that the product will prevent such and such diseases. (I call this the fear tactic.)

3) **Ingredient List "As-Long-As-Your-Arm"**: marketers load products with a broad array of nutrients, including vitamins, minerals, nutraceuticals, digestive aids, and herbs so that the label looks like the food and wine shopping list for a weekend-long party for 100 people. (This is also known as the "if this product contains all these incredible nutrients in one capsule, it must be good for you" tactic.)

False Claims

I have designed a supplement that meets the criteria for the proper design of a supplement to meet your daily needs for all essential nutrients. There are two jars: one for minerals and one for vitamins. The recommended dose is 8 capsules per day for <u>each</u> product—that's 16 capsules per day! And this product *meets* your needs and contains the finest ingredients on earth.

I recently saw a TV infomercial that marketed a supplement that the manufacturer claimed was the finest product in the world. The recommended dose was 4 capsules per day. Now, I spared no expense to design my product, and cost was never a consideration. I designed the product to the exacting requirements as outlined in this monograph. I *did not* limit myself to a pre-conceived price that was compatible with a consumer's budget; I wanted primarily to meet the consumer's nutritional needs.

My daily dose is 16 capsules per day. The "best supplement in the world" requires the use of only 4 capsules per day. Why the difference? It's simple. They're lying! The product uses inferior ingredients (they say it uses the best), the quantities for some nutrients are less than needed (calcium and magnesium specifically), and the antioxidants are mostly carotenoids (the **Second Line of Defense**).

The product contains no vitamin Q which is the most important (and expensive antioxidant). It sells for $29.95 for a one-month supply. My product costs more than that just to manufacture!

The minute you enter the price-competitive mass market, you need large margins for everyone in the chain-of-profit to make money. Mark-ups in the supplement business are 5-10 times: example, the cost of goods is $3.00, and the selling price is $30.00 (10 times mark-up).

For TV marketing, you need, at least, a 7-10 times mark-up— minimum! There is no other way; these are the numbers. So the whole marketing program for "the best supplement in the world" is a lie. For them to sell this product at $29.95 means that the cost for manufacturing it must be no higher than $4.25. It cannot possibly contain the finest ingredients, in the right amount, to meet your nutritional requirements!

Review the section on minerals to see how many capsules it takes to meet your nutrient needs when you use the right ingredients; it cannot be done in 4 capsules!

I formulated my supplement and I contracted with a company to buy the raw materials, put them into capsules, package the capsules into a bottle, and finally to place a label on the jar. I do the marketing directly to the end user: there are no middlemen, no distributors, and no brokers, each taking a piece of the pie. That's why I can provide you with the truly best product at a price no one else can match. There are no other hands in the pie.

Fear Tactic

Using the second technique, a nutritional supplement company may have from 5 to 30 (or more) different products in their company product line. And the slick naming of the product adds to the confusion. For example, product names, such as **Brain Elixir**, **Kidney Tonic**, **Joint Relief**, **Body Energizer**, **Formula for Bone Health**, **Formula for Diabetes**, **Eye Formula**, and **Formula for Heart Health**, all suggest a specific purpose provided by the nutritional supplements in a particular bottle.

Yet, despite of the claim that each bottle provides a unique formulation for that specific condition, each bottle often contains many of the same individual nutritional supplements. Remember, there are only about 30 <u>essential</u> nutrients that our bodies need each day. So, what the companies do is mix and match these essential nutrients, using a shotgun approach. For example, people who suffer from asthma have been shown to have a deficiency of vitamin B6 and magnesium. Therefore, the focus of the design for an Asthma Formula will, very likely, include at least these two nutrients along with other nutrients such as herbs or other nutraceuticals that might work with this condition.

The major problem with this strategy is that the combination, or additive effect of, the nutrients contained within each individual product may provide a daily dose of a specific nutrient that is above the safe level. In the other instance, depending on how many different supplements one takes each day, the use of the product may lead to a very high dose of some nutrients and, at the same time, a very low dose of some other essential nutrients.

Or, even worse, one may use five or more different products whose formulations contain only some of the essential nutrients. The downside to this is that one may seriously unbalance his nutritional status and, also, possibly end up with a serious nutritional deficiency because the manufacturer did not include several of the essential nutrients in the formulations.

This will lead to a significant disruption in the homeostasis or balance of the internal environment of the body. One cannot take a casual attitude toward nutritional supplementation; I have stressed this theme throughout this monograph. Many people actually form an emotional attachment to the supplement program and, like any addiction, they continue to use more and more without having any idea of the impact of this supplement misuse on the health of their body.

Another strong marketing strategy is to pitch a specific formula for people of different ages and of different sexes. In this strategy, there is a multi-vitamin and mineral formula for **Senior Men** and **Senior Women**, **Adult Men** and **Adult Women**, **Teens: Male** and **Female Formulas**, and a **Prenatal Formula**. And on it goes until one runs out of population groups for which to develop yet another specialized formulation!

Returning to the charts presented earlier in this monograph and the abundant amount of scientific research regarding the nutritional needs of humans, we find that we all need, essentially, the same 30 nutrients each day in our daily diet, with only minor variations in the amount of nutrients we consume.

In general, the main variation is based primarily on body size: the bigger you are, the more you need within certain limitations that can easily be determined by using the above-mentioned charts. I have studied the labels of these population-based formulations and their listed content of nutrients. The formulations are, in general, very similar: there are few differences in the ingredient contents among the different product formulas.

Reviewing the list of essential nutrients, which may number 20 to 30 different nutrient items, one finds that the majority of them are identical in quantity. The difference between two brands may be that one formula has 100 milligrams more of magnesium and the other, 100 IU more of vitamin D. There is absolutely no scientific rationale to make these very minor changes in the formulation.

The only logical conclusion that I can draw is that the variations in the formula enable the formulator to create a market niche and brand loyalty by providing the user with a false sense of security that this product was developed specifically for his needs. Nothing could be further from the truth.

Also in the realm of specific formulas aimed at increasing the efficacy of a particular nutritional supplement is the gimmick of **AM/PM** administration of a nutrient complex. This protocol suggests that some nutrients are better absorbed from the intestinal tract and incorporated into the cells when administered at one time, or another, of the day. Next, I suspect that these paragons of scientific research will tell us that we can eat eggs only in the morning and meat only at night because the necessary digestive processes for these individual foods are time related.

The absurdity of these ideas should be apparent without any further elaboration from me. And, any suggestion to the contrary, invoking support from scientific literature, is even more compelling evidence of a manufacturer's attempt to slip his hand into your wallet and cleanly extract your money.

Ingredient List "As-Long-As-Your-Arm" Technique

The third technique used by product formulators to deceive the public is the technique of adding so many different ingredients to the formula that the list is "as-long-as-your-arm." In all cases, most of the ingredients listed are nowhere near a therapeutic dose; the sole purpose of adding a pinch of this and a pinch of that is to impress the potential consumer with how many hot or powerful ingredients are contained within the supplement.

For example, one product that I recently reviewed, called **Advanced Antioxidant Complex**, contained vitamin Q (CoQ10) in a daily dosage level of 10 mg. I have previously described the adequate daily dose for CoQ10, and 10 mg doesn't cut it. In the same formula, 10 mg of lipoic acid was listed on the label, but a therapeutic dose of lipoic acid is about 600 mg per day.

Both items are very expensive, so instead of designing a therapeutic formula containing the appropriate amount of these nutrients, the formulator decided that he would dupe the potential consumer who, in general, has little knowledge or understanding about how much of the nutrient is required to meet his needs. To formulate a product, using these nutrients in the appropriate quantities, requires more than one-half of a double-0 capsule to meet your needs.

Now imagine: The recommended dose is three capsules per day for the *total* multi-vitamin and mineral product, which also contains, theoretically, a therapeutic dose of vitamin Q and lipoic acid. I have already shown you the capsule size necessary to meet daily quantitative vitamin and mineral requirements. Do you really think that this manufacturer's product can actually do what it advertises? No way!

Another product that is part of the **Advanced Antioxidant**

77

Complex formulation has a chef's-stew of phytochemicals (herbs), none of which meets the quantity requirements for therapeutic action. So the unsuspecting consumer, thrilled at the label-bursting number of nutrients contained within the formulation, hands over his hard-earned money (again), receiving little value for his investment.

This format of product design is rampant throughout the nutritional supplement industry. I urge you not to be deceived. With knowledge, you'll discover that it is not complicated to make a right choice for the supplements that you use.

The first requirement is to choose a formulation that contains all of the essential nutrients. Do not get caught-up in the hype over nutraceuticals—these are not essential nutrients. If you choose to use any of the newer, modern-day nutraceuticals, choose them carefully based on your knowledge of the ones that may be effective and beneficial to your health.

Always keep in mind the distinction between the essential nutrients (the 30 or so vitamins and minerals that you need each day to be healthy) and the group of nutrients that are not essential to your health. This is the nutraceutical group and it contains the many hundreds of other nutrients lining the shelves of the nutritional supplement marketing machines.

Discussion of the use of nutraceuticals is beyond the scope of this monograph. Only the essential nutrients concern us. They provide the basic core nutrients that are the foundation of your supplementation program. Nutraceuticals, including non-essential vitamins, herbs, and other newly synthesized non-vitamin/non-mineral nutrients, must take a backseat to the essential nutrients.

Your best choice is a multi-vitamin and mineral supplement that contains all of the essential nutrients in their most absorbed form, manufactured from the best possible chemical sources. Make sure that the nutrients are in the correct balance and proportion to maximize the health benefits you hope to derive from their use.

I believe that you are now prepared, and armed, to meet the enemy: these are the marketers of supplements who want only to extract the money from your wallet but offer you little in return for your investment and even less toward the improvement of your health. Good hunting.

Dr. Gregory S. Ellis, PhD
Certified Nutrition Specialist

11 Nutrients: Functions and Food Sources

What You Need	What It Does	Food Source
Vitamin A	prevents night blindness, forms and maintains healthy skin, hair, nails, and mucous membranes; fights infections	milk, egg yolks, organ meats, leafy green vegetables, broccoli, carrots, pumpkin, apricots
Vitamin B1 (thiamin)	helps convert food to energy; promotes proper nerve function, appetite, and digestion	pork, beef, enriched breads and cereals, nuts, sunflower seeds, soybeans
Vitamin B2 (riboflavin)	helps to convert food to energy; keeps skin healthy	milk, cheese, yogurt, enriched bread and cereals, broccoli, almonds, liver
Niacin	provides energy in body cells, assists in nerve function	peanuts, meat, poultry, fish, breads and cereal
Vitamin B6	maintains nervous system; helps fight infection, rearranges amino acids	meat, poultry, fish, whole-grain cereals, wheat germ, nuts, beans, bananas
Pantothenate	release of energy from carbohydrates and fats, builds steroid hormones	meat, poultry, legumes, whole-grain cereals
Vitamin B12	keeps blood healthy, acts as a co-enzyme in cell metabolism	dairy products, meat, fish
Folic acid	important during pregnancy, maintains cell division and growth	spinach and other leafy green vegetables, avocados, brewers yeast, and oranges

What You Need	What It Does	Food Source
Vitamin C	keeps teeth and gums healthy, promotes healing, helps fight infections, assists in collagen formation	citrus fruits like oranges, strawberries, broccoli, cabbage, tomatoes, and potatoes
Vitamin D	helps form and maintain strong bones and teeth, aids in absorbing calcium	milk and dairy products, sunlight, and egg yolks
Vitamin E	helps form and maintain blood cells, muscles, and other tissues	vegetable oils, green leafy vegetables, butter, margarine, wheat germ
Calcium	helps build and maintain strong bones and teeth, acts in muscle and nerve function, assists in blood clotting	milk, cheese, yogurt, soy products, broccoli
Iron	transports oxygen to cells, maintains healthy blood	lean red meat, fish, poultry, breads and cereals, leafy green vegetables
Manganese	involved in enzyme systems and antioxidant reactions	whole grains and cereal products, some fruits and vegetables
Copper	promotes healthy blood and heart function, acts in enzyme systems, important in bone and nerve structure	organ meats, seafood, nuts, and seeds
Chromium	blood glucose (blood sugar) and fat metabolism	cheese, calf liver, wheat germ
Zinc	regulates immune system, promotes normal taste and vision, speeds wound healing	lean meat, poultry, fish, whole grains, beans, peas, nuts, seafood, cheese

Table 12.

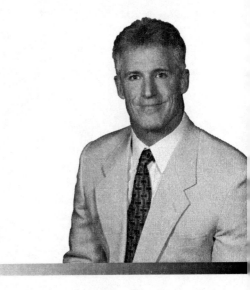

About the Author

Dr. Gregory Ellis received his Ph.D. degree from the Temple University School of Medicine's Department of Physiology. He has a graduate level certification in nutrition from the American College of Nutrition (Certified Nutrition Specialist). In the early 1970's he opened one of the first Nautilus exercise centers in the country. He has consulted with professional and amateur athletes. He has an extensive knowledge of weight control and muscle building and has completed pioneering research in body composition. He specializes in the biochemistry of energy metabolism and nutritional supplementation. Dr. Ellis believes in integrating research with its ultimate goal: application for use by individuals.

In addition to lecturing and writing, Dr. Ellis has developed cutting-edge nutritional products, exercise equipment, and monitoring devices for weight control and fitness. His extensive knowledge in so many varied areas about health improvement and fitness is unique. Dr. Ellis operates a large clinical nutrition practice in the suburban Philadelphia area.